The Depression Helpbook

Wayne Katon, M.D.   PSYCHIATRIST
Evette Ludman Ph.D.   PSYCHOLOGIST
Gregory E. Simon, M.D., M.P.H.   PSYCHIATRIST
Elizabeth Lin, M.D., M.P.H.   FAMILY PHYSICIAN
Michael Von Korff, Sc.D.   HEALTH SCIENCES RESEARCH
Edward Walker, M.D.   PSYCHIATRIST
Mark Sullivan, M.D., Ph.D.   PSYCHIATRIST
Terry Bush, Ph.D.   PSYCHOLOGIST
Louise Carter, Ph.D.   HEALTH WRITER

GROUP HEALTH COOPERATIVE CENTER FOR HEALTH STUDIES
UNIVERSITY OF WASHINGTON, DEPARTMENT OF PSYCHIATRY

BULL PUBLISHING COMPANY
BOULDER, COLORADO

Published by Bull Publishing Company, Post Office Box 1377, Boulder, Colorado 80306 (www.bullpub.com)

Library of Congress Cataloging-in-Publication Data
The depression helpbook / by Wayne Katon . . . [et al.].
    p. cm.
Includes index.
    ISBN 0-923521-68-2
1. Depression, Mental—Treatment. 2. Depression, Mental—Alternative
treatment. I. Katon, Wayne.
    RC537.D4278 2002
    616.85'2706—dc21   2002001970

ACKNOWLEDGMENTS

The authors' work in preparing and evaluating this book was supported by a grant from the National Institute of Mental Health (R01-MH41739). All royalties from the sale of this book will be used for continued research on improving care for depression.

The authors wish to acknowledge the work of Peter Lewinsohn, colleagues, and former students. Much of this work is based on the Coping with Depression Course and its adaptation for adolescents. Some of the material on relaxation and assertiveness skills has been adapted from the work of Susan Curry and colleagues at the Group Health Cooperative Center for Health Studies.

Jessica Ridpath provided invaluable editorial assistance.

CONTENTS

How to Use This Book

GOALS

This book is for people with chronic or recurrent depression. Studies show that most people with depression have recurrent depression—meaning their symptoms come back again. Some people have depression that lasts for several years. Doctors call this chronic depression. The goals of this book are to help you

- Develop confidence in your ability to manage your depression, even when it is severe

- Achieve and maintain balance in your mood and your life when you start to feel better

- Reduce the chance that your depression will come back

Many people who experience recurrent or repeated episodes of depression have learned how to manage their condition. Some take medications to prevent a relapse. Others rely on counseling or behavioral changes that have worked in the past. It's also common for people to mix and match, using a combination of medication and therapy. Regardless of your approach, the strategy that you are applying is known as **self care**, a term that you will encounter many times in this book. Self care refers to the things you can do for yourself. But it does not mean you're on your own. An essential part of self care is the partnership you have with your doctor and other health care professionals. There is no simple formula for treating depression. While people with depression can benefit from the strategies in this book, other treatments are also available. It is important for you to work with your doctor to find out what is best for you.

ABOUT THIS BOOK

This book was written by a team of psychiatrists, psychologists, and primary care physicians who have worked with thousands of people coping with depression. In these pages, the results of research studies and the opinions of experts are supplemented with the words of real people who have experienced depression. Tapping all of these sources makes it possible to present the best available information on how to achieve balance in your mood and your life, manage depression day by day, and reduce the chances of severe recurrence.

This book is organized into brief chapters. Each contains essential information about a particular aspect of managing depression. There is also a chapter written specifically for your family and friends, should you care to share this book with them. Additional resources are listed at the back of the book.

You do not have to read this book from cover to cover. You may want to read the first few introductory chapters and then skip to other chapters that interest you most.

BE PATIENT

Just as depression usually does not appear overnight, learning to control and prevent depression takes time. If there were quick fixes, fewer people would be affected by recurrent or persistent bouts of depression.

If you have difficulty with a technique recommended in this book, remember that doing something new often requires several tries and that your progress may be gradual. As you experiment, stick with a particular technique for 3 or 4 weeks to give it a chance to work. Don't give up too soon! People close to you may notice an improvement in your mood or your behavior before you do. Be on the lookout for small positive changes. They can be significant and may give you the boost you need to get yourself back on track.

Part I

A BETTER UNDERSTANDING

What to Expect in This Section

A better understanding of

- How depression can affect you
- What causes depression
- How to get started on the path to recovery

FACT
Approximately 10% of adults will at some point experience a depressive episode that would benefit from treatment. —*Scientific American Medicine*

FAMOUS PEOPLE WITH DEPRESSION
Ludwig van Beethoven, Charles Dickens, Patty Duke, Vivian Leigh, Abraham Lincoln, Eugene O'Neill, Virginia Wolf

---

CHAPTER 1

What Is Depression?

I had been having trouble sleeping and was tired all the time. It was getting harder and harder to keep up with my responsibilities at work because I couldn't concentrate. I felt people didn't want to be around me because I was gloomy and irritable. My physical health seemed to have taken a turn for the worse, which had me down in the dumps. So I went to see my doctor. When he asked if I was depressed, it took me completely by surprise.

HOW TO RECOGNIZE DEPRESSION

Depression is a medical condition that is both physical and psychological. The primary symptoms are feelings of sorrow, dejection, despair, or irritability. Most people feel sad or blue occasionally, but when these feelings persist or worsen and begin to interfere with work or personal relationships, depression is suspected.

Learning how to identify depression in its early stages is important. Many people, even those who have been treated for depression in the past, don't realize that they are depressed (or that they're slipping back into a depression) until their depression is severe. If you can recognize depression when it first begins to come on, it is often much easier to manage.

Many of the symptoms of depression, such as headache, backache, or stomach trouble, are physical and may come on gradually, so it's often hard to recognize that depression is developing. A good way to find out is to review the Symptom Checklist for Recognizing Depression (opposite page). If you have been experiencing five or more of the symptoms on this list most of the time for at least 2 weeks, then depression is a likely explanation.

DEPRESSION IS COMMON

You probably know people who have been depressed in the past or several who are struggling with depression right now. Even highly accomplished and famous people experience depression from time to time. Television journalist Mike Wallace, President Abraham Lincoln, British Prime

SYMPTOM CHECKLIST FOR RECOGNIZING DEPRESSION

_____ Feeling sad, blue, irritable, or tearful

_____ Trouble sleeping or sleeping too much

_____ Fatigue or loss of energy

_____ Feeling slowed down _or_ restless and unable to sit still

_____ Changes in appetite or weight loss or gain

_____ Loss of interest in activities you normally enjoy, such as sex

_____ Feeling worthless or guilty

_____ Feeling pessimistic or hopeless

_____ Problems concentrating or thinking

_____ Thoughts of death or suicide

_____ Aches and pains such as headache, stomachache, back pain

_____ Increased anxiety and tension or anxiety attacks

Minister Winston Churchill, and award-winning author William Styron are just a few of the well-known people who have battled depression.

Even so, when you're the one who's depressed, you often feel isolated. You may hesitate to tell others about your depression. Or, feeling that you should be able to overcome this illness on your own, you may wait to seek help until your depression becomes severe. Remember that depression is very common. One out of every four women and nearly one in seven men will suffer from at least one depressive episode sometime during their life.

WHAT CAUSES DEPRESSION?

Experts now believe that depression is due to a combination of biological susceptibility and major life stresses. Depression tends to run in families, just like other medical conditions, such as diabetes, asthma, and hypertension, so depression probably has a genetic component, as do these other diseases. People who suffer from depression seem to have inherited a heightened sensitivity to changes in the levels of certain chemicals in the brain.

For some people, no specific event leads to their initial depression. For many others, certain experiences can trigger their first depressive episodes. It may be a painful physical illness or a traumatic event.

Major life stresses, such as divorce or death of a loved one, as well as positive changes like starting a new job, moving to another city, or having a new baby, can reduce the availability of key chemical messengers in the brain. These chemical messengers, called neurotransmitters, regulate sleep, energy, appetite, motivation, mood, and the ability to experience pleasure, to think, and to concentrate. For people who experience repeated episodes of depression, or who feel depressed most of the time, stress is more likely to lead to reductions in the levels of these chemicals.

DEPRESSION IS TREATABLE

When these essential chemical messengers are replenished, depressed people generally start to feel better. One way to restore these brain chemicals is by taking antidepressant medication. Another way is psychotherapy that treats depression by helping patients to improve their relationships with others, develop more constructive ways of thinking, and increase participation in more pleasant and rewarding activities. Psychotherapy is often combined with antidepressant medication.

Some people think they should be able to cope with depression on their own, without medications, psychotherapy, or any kind of outside help. But bear in mind that no one expects people with asthma or diabetes to overcome their illnesses simply by doing a better job of managing stress. The same should be true for depression. As soon as you recognize the problem, it makes sense to get help.

For people who experience repeated episodes of depression, long-term use of prescription antidepressant medicine can help prevent severe recurrences of the disease. Making the decision to use medication to combat depression is not a sign of weakness. Many people find that long-term use of antidepressants helps them feel and cope better day to day and prevents recurrences of severe depression. Taking medication may be an important part of your self-care and a sign that you are willing to do what works for you.

EVERYBODY'S DEPRESSION IS DIFFERENT

Each person who experiences depression is different, so it's not surprising that people with depression don't all experience it in the same way. The symptoms that bother you the most may not be so troubling for someone else.

People also differ in the circumstances that bring on depression. Sometimes depression occurs after a sudden stressful event such as a failed love affair, an illness, the loss of a job, or the death of someone close. Even positive events like getting a promotion can bring on depression.

Depression can result from long-term pressures: a difficult marriage, a stressful job or a chronic illness. In some cases, depression comes on after what seems like a minor event, or even for no reason at all.

Chuck's story:

I started getting depressed around age 12. I missed 20 to 30 days of school a semester from junior high through high school. But I didn't realize what was wrong, so I didn't start getting help until I was 30 years old. I didn't want to admit I needed help. I wanted to do it myself.

Janet's story:

I was kind of relieved when the doctor said my problem was depression because I thought something was really wrong. Depression affects my colon, my gut—and that worried me because my dad died of cancer and I have lots of cancer in my family. But when I thought about what the doctor said, I realized that, yes, I am depressed.

Stanley's story:

Everything was going wrong. I was under a lot of stress. My shoulders started aching, and I got muscle spasms across my back. There was no reason for it. I'm usually very positive, but I wasn't being rational. I noticed I wasn't getting things done.

Types Of Depression

Depressions also differ in how severe they are, how long they last, and what the symptoms are. Each type of depression belongs to a specific category. Knowing the category helps guide medical professionals in recommending the right treatment.

Major depression consists of at least five symptoms on the checklist at the beginning of this chapter, such as sleep problems or feeling worthless, for 2 or more weeks.

Minor depression includes some depressive symptoms, but not enough to count as major depression. Sometimes minor depression continues after the worst part of a major depressive episode has passed.

Dysthymia is what mental health professionals call a chronic depression that may be less severe, but lasts for 2 years or longer. People with dysthymia often report that they have struggled with depressive moods for most of their lives.

Manic depression (also called manic-depressive illness or bipolar disorder) is a rarer form in which people suffer periods of major depression alternating with periods of exuberance and high energy. During the exuberant phases, people who are manic-depressive experience euphoria, extraordinary vigor, and increased talkativeness and sociability. They may also do unusually risky or impulsive things. Manic depression requires different kinds of treatment from those described in this book.

Consult the Resource Guide at the back of this book for sources of further information on manic depression.

HOW LONG WILL MY DEPRESSION LAST?

Don't delay getting help for depression because you hope it will go away on its own. Left untreated, a major depressive episode usually lasts 6–9 months, although one out of three depressed people do feel better after about 3 months, even without treatment.

Both antidepressant medications and the specific psychotherapies described in this book speed up the time to recovery. With medication, most people improve significantly in 2–4 weeks, and with psychotherapy, in 6–8 weeks. It is important to continue taking your antidepressant medication and attending psychotherapy sessions for as long as you and your doctor think necessary, even if you are feeling much better.

What If I Am Prone To Chronic Depression?

Controlling depression may be more difficult for people who are particularly vulnerable because of their genetic makeup or their childhood experiences. The tools described in this book (including antidepressant medications, developing more constructive ways of thinking, increasing positive activities, and improving interactions with others) can help anyone struggling to manage depression.

CHAPTER 2

Reversing the Downward Spiral of Depression

About 6 weeks ago I got into a terrible accident. Afterward, my neck and back were really stiff and always hurting, and I couldn't sleep. I was really tired and couldn't concentrate on my work. I could tell that my boss was getting ticked off, but he didn't come out and say so. I avoided him any chance I could get. I used to play soccer after work, but now I would just go home and collapse on the couch. I was getting really irritable with my wife and kids, and then my wife got upset because I wasn't pulling my weight around the house. That's when I started to feel really down. My life was spinning out of control, and I didn't seem able to do anything about it.

DEPRESSION CAUSES A DOWNWARD SPIRAL

Depression affects the whole person. It influences your physical well-being, your thoughts and your feelings. People who are depressed usually stop doing things they once enjoyed, like talking to friends or getting projects done around the house. They also begin to have doubts about whether they can succeed in those things.

Depression can feed upon itself, making you feel worse and worse. For example, if you stop doing things you enjoy, you become unhappy. If you're unhappy, you might spend more time alone, which may make you feel depressed. As a result, you become less active and feel even more depressed—and so on. This cycle of worsening depression is sometimes called a *negative downward spiral* (Figure 2-1).

How does the spiral start? It's different for different people. Sometimes stressful events such as work or family problems can trigger a downward spiral. Physical problems such as chronic pain (headaches, backaches), insomnia, or lack or energy can also begin a spiral of depressed feelings. Persistent negative thought patterns or becoming less active or productive are other initial steps in a negative downward spiral.

REVERSING THE DOWNWARD SPIRAL

The good news is that it's possible to break a cycle of worsening depression and turn a negative spiral into a *positive upward spiral* (Figure 2-2). Taking an antidepressant can

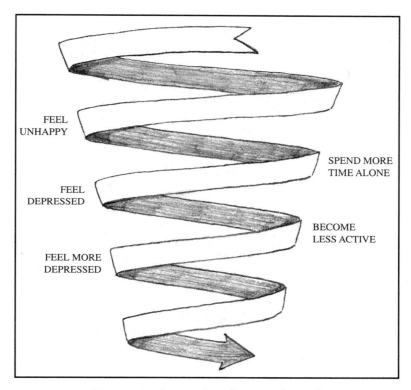

FEEL
UNHAPPY

SPEND MORE
TIME ALONE

FEEL
DEPRESSED

BECOME
LESS ACTIVE

FEEL MORE
DEPRESSED

Figure 2-1—A negative downward spiral

help you begin a positive spiral. These medications restore your energy so that you'll feel like engaging in fun and rewarding activities. They can also restore normal sleep and decrease physical pain. Other strategies that can help you reverse the negative spiral of depression include

- Doing things you enjoy
- Putting a positive spin on your thinking

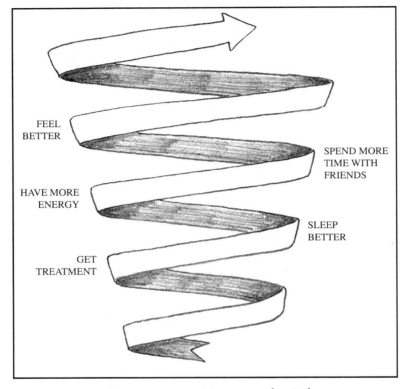

Figure 2-2—A positive upward spiral

- Improving your relationships with friends and family
- Exercising regularly
- Establishing a regular sleep pattern

Some of these sound simple, but when you're depressed it can take a lot of effort to get involved in any activity—even if you think it will make you less depressed.

Taking that first step to do something for yourself is often the hardest part. But it's worth the effort to reverse your downward spiral and start moving in an upward, positive direction again.

When I told my doctor about the problems I was having, he said he thought I had become depressed. He explained that injuries can lead to fatigue and demoralization that could bring on depression. Pain and injury can also make you stop doing fun things and make you irritable. He had me pegged! So he prescribed an antidepressant, and that helped me to sleep better right away. After a few weeks, my wife said that I seemed to have more energy and that I was less cranky and negative. I began to follow through on all those things that had piled up at work and around the house. I even went to soccer. As I began to do things again, I noticed that I felt better about myself. Best of all, I began to feel more in control.

CHAPTER 3

Making Your Own Decision About Treatment

After being laid off from my job, I began to feel blue, to worry about finances, and my energy and concentration both decreased. I started to exercise regularly and to schedule activities with friends since that usually helps improve my mood. But over the next month, I began to have trouble sleeping and I was so tired all the time, so I decided to see my doctor about antidepressant medication or counseling.

HOW TO KNOW WHEN SELF-CARE ISN'T ENOUGH

Good self-care is a central part of getting and staying well. For everyone who suffers from depression, developing and practicing the self-care skills described in Part 2 of this book is a good first step. Sometimes, though, good self-care alone is not enough. In some cases, it may be clear in the beginning that treatment for depression is necessary. In other situations, you may decide to see a doctor or other professional about treatment if significant problems with depression persist despite your best self-care efforts. Depression which is more severe and more persistent (what doctors and therapists call *major depression*) is less likely to resolve completely with self-care alone—and more likely to need some professional treatment.

WHAT ARE YOUR TREATMENT OPTIONS

Several treatments for depression have been proven effective and safe. Treatment of depression is successful as often as (or more often than) treatment of most other significant health problems. Effective treatments include several types of psychotherapy specifically developed to treat depression as well as several effective antidepressant medications (more than 20 at the time this book was written). Before making a decision, you should take some time to consider these various options. This chapter includes some advice on how to make an informed decision. Chapters 5 and 6 of this book include specific information about the various options available.

WHAT TO CONSIDER AND WHAT TO IGNORE

Consider Your Previous Experience

You may have some experience with treatment of depression—either medications or psychotherapy. If a type of treatment was very helpful in the past, it is likely to be helpful again. For example, an antidepressant medication that was very effective and caused no side effects would probably be a good choice the second time around. If a particular treatment (a specific medication, a specific psychotherapist) was not helpful in the past, you might want to try a different option this time. There are plenty of effective options available. If a particular treatment was not helpful before, however, you shouldn't write off all similar treatments. If your earlier experience with one psychotherapist or type of psychotherapy was a negative one, a different therapist or type of therapy might still be very helpful. The same rule applies to different antidepressant medications.

Consider (Somewhat) the Experience of Friends and Relatives

It's often helpful to discuss your situation with family or friends. It's likely that some of them have had treatment for depression in the past, and they might have some useful advice. Try, however, to not be too strongly influenced by one person's negative experience. Every individual is different, and someone else's experience with a particular treatment (medication or psychotherapy) may not apply at all to you. Think of what you'd do before buying a particular kind of car. You'd probably ask for advice from one or two people who own one—but you'd probably also read one of the consumer magazines to see if their experience was typical.

Consider the Evidence

Just as you'd read one of the consumer magazines before buying a car, you should consider what research says about various treatments for depression. Research on treatment does just what the consumer magazines do—it considers the average experience of large groups of people. It's true that each average is made up of many individuals with different experiences, but a description of the average effectiveness of treatment is a good place to start. The following chapters in this book describe what research says about the pros and cons of various treatments for depression.

Consider the Practical Issues

There are several practical issues that can make a particular treatment more or less likely to work out for you: how much it will cost you, how far you'll have to travel, whether the treatment is available at a time convenient for you. Try to find out about these things before you make a decision. Any treatment for depression (medication or psychotherapy) is likely to involve several visits over a few months. You're less likely to stick with (and benefit from) a treatment which is too expensive or inconvenient.

Ignore Any Ideas About What Getting Treatment "Means"

It's only natural to wonder about the "meaning" of depression or the "meaning" of getting treatment. Unfortunately, this wondering often gets in the way of getting help. For example, you may think that taking medication for depression (or seeing a therapist) means that you've "lost control" or that you "can't handle life." In fact, getting treatment for depression doesn't mean any more than getting treatment for any other medical problem. We don't wonder what it "means" when someone gets treatment for high blood pressure or asthma. We do wonder, however, when someone won't consider treatment that can really help.

Ignore Guilt and Prejudice

Exaggerated or irrational negative ideas are a central part of depression. Unfortunately, these ideas can get in the way of getting the help you need. Feelings of guilt or shame can make it hard to ask anyone for help. You may worry about what others will think. You may feel that you don't deserve to feel any better than you do. All of these thoughts, of course, are just the depression talking. You should consider several factors in making your decision about treatment but try not to consider these guilty or self-critical thoughts at all.

WHAT ARE YOUR FIRST IMPRESSIONS?

At this point you may have some first impressions about various treatment options. These impressions could be based on what you've read, your own previous experience, or what you've heard from others. It's a good idea to write these down. Your final decision may be very different from any first impression, but recording your thoughts now can help you to identify questions you have and areas you want to know more about. Writing down your thoughts about treatment can also help you to see if any of them fall into the category of reasons you should try to ignore.

First impressions about antidepressant medication:

PROs

1. _____

2. _____

3. _____

CONs

1._____

2._____

3._____

First impressions about psychotherapy for depression:

PROs

1. _____

2. _____

3. _____

CONs

1. _____

2. _____

3. _____

Before you read further, take a few minutes to look over your list. Do any of your reasons fall into the category of reasons you'd be better off ignoring? If so, scratch them out. Which areas do you need to know more about? We encourage you to read Chapters 4, 5, and 6 before making your decision about what to do next.

CHAPTER 4

Working with Your Doctor

Seeing my doctor made me nervous. For some reason, I would clam up whenever I got into the doctor's office. Finally, I started writing notes to myself about my symptoms and my concerns. During my next visit, I took my notes in and discussed them with the doctor.

GETTING HELP

Finding effective treatment for depression often starts with a visit to a health professional who specializes in primary care, typically a physician, nurse practitioner, or physician assistant. You know that fluctuations in mood are a normal part of life, but you may not be sure how to distinguish between ordinary sadness and depression that's serious enough to warrant medical treatment or counseling. Talking with your doctor can help you decide.

Choosing a Doctor

Doctors frequently help patients deal with depression. The key is to choose one who makes you feel comfortable when discussing your problems and who is skilled in diagnosing and treating depression. If after talking to your doctor you don't feel confident that the two of you can form a partnership to manage your depression, you may want to try someone else.

COMMUNICATING WITH YOUR DOCTOR

Talking with your doctor isn't always easy. The two of you may sometimes have different ideas about what's important. You may be nervous, or you may worry that you have a serious medical problem but feel afraid to ask about it. Maybe you want to discuss something but feel embarrassed to bring it up. Or you may be convinced that you'll never feel better. Many people feel their doctor is always in a hurry and doesn't have enough time for them.

Four steps can be taken to prevent communication problems between you and your doctor:

1. Come prepared
2. Ask questions
3. Discuss problems
4. Ask for educational materials

The following patient stories, which illustrate common problems, will help make these four points clearer.

1. COME PREPARED

Ellen's story:

I started having headaches at work, felt tired, and couldn't get anything done. One day I had an especially bad headache, so I made an appointment to see a doctor. When she asked what the problem was, all I could think of was that I wanted to get rid of my headache. After she examined me and asked me some more questions, she told me that my headache could be due to tension and suggested that over-the-counter pain relievers and relaxation exercises might help. I left the office feeling discouraged because I had already tried acetaminophen and aspirin, and they hadn't helped. And how could I get relaxed when I had these headaches all the time?

Ellen's visit with the doctor might have been more successful had she come prepared to describe her whole pattern of symptoms. In addition to talking about that morning's headache, she could have mentioned that she always felt tired, frustrated, and unable to complete tasks on time. She should also have explained that she had already tried pain relievers without success.

It's difficult to come up with an organized, concise message when you're in pain. One way around this difficulty is to make a list of symptoms and questions as they occur to you before you go to the doctor. Refer to your notes during the visit. It also helps to have a clear objective of what you want to achieve by the end of the visit.

2. ASK QUESTIONS

Jill's story:
My doctor referred me to counseling after diagnosing my depression. I couldn't understand how talking to a counselor could help, so I delayed going. When I went back for my headaches, I finally asked. My doctor explained how counseling could provide me with tools, such as relaxation exercises and other ways of reducing stress, that might help me concentrate better on my studies.

To help forge an effective partnership, Jill's doctor should have encouraged questions. Jill could have helped herself by telling her doctor that she didn't understand how counseling might help her.

Don't be afraid to carry a pen and notepad so that you can write down the things that are being said during the visit. Questions may pop into your mind on the way home or after discussing things with your partner, family member, or friend.

3. DISCUSS PROBLEMS

Scott's story: *After I started taking an antidepressant, I began to have headaches and felt lightheaded. So I stopped taking the pills. When my doctor asked how my depression was, I didn't want to disappoint him, so I only said that the medicine wasn't working. My doctor suggested increasing the dose.*

The doctor should have encouraged Scott to mention any problems with the medication. Scott's problems might also have been resolved more quickly if he had called the doctor for advice rather than stopping the medication on his own.

If you have taken antidepressant medication in the past, be sure to tell your doctor which ones have worked for you and which ones have not. If you know of a medication that has helped a family member with depression, mention this as well.

4. ASK FOR READING MATERIALS

Phyllis' story:

My doctor explained that depression could be causing my sleeplessness and fatigue, and suggested that being more

active and taking antidepressant medication might help me.
But I still felt confused. I would have liked for the doctor to
explain things again, but I knew there were other patients
waiting, so I left.

Phyllis could have asked if there were any reading materials that would help her understand her depression better. Her doctor might have given her a book to take home. Some doctors also have a list of reading materials, many of them available at no cost at the public library.

Your doctor may be able to supply a list of depression support groups, which are also excellent sources of information. If not, you can find the names, addresses, and phone numbers of several depression support groups in the Resource Guide at the back of this book.

WHAT ARE YOUR OPTIONS?

If either you or your doctor thinks you could benefit from a more specialized program or from counseling, referral to a mental health specialist might be a good idea.

In some circumstances, you may choose to go outside your health plan for specialized care. For example, you may want a second opinion. Or your health plan may not cover the particular treatment or therapist you prefer. In these situations, keep in mind that you may have to pay the full cost of your treatment. If you are not in a managed care plan, you should check with your provider regarding your coverage. There is often a limit on yearly mental health care coverage.

If your insurance plan doesn't cover the cost of counseling and you can't afford it on your own, you should explore other options. Your doctor should be able to supply you with information about community-sponsored or low-cost counseling programs—and also about depression support groups. You'll also find a list of depression support groups at the end of this book. These groups know a lot about coping with depression and can be excellent sources of information about treatment options.

DEVELOPING A PLAN TOGETHER

Your plan for managing depression is likely to include changes in your lifestyle and, in many cases, prescription antidepressant medicine as well. Your doctor may give you specific suggestions on how to deal with your problems and encourage activities that make you feel better. He or she may also focus on adjusting the dosage of your antidepressant. When you start feeling better consistently, you will not need to see your doctor so often. But if you have concerns or problems, call the office or write them down for your next visit. Do not stop taking your medicine without first having a discussion with your health care provider.

What If You Have Additional Questions?

Ask them. It's common to have new questions once you get home. For example, you may have thought you knew all you needed to know when your doctor explained how an antidepressant worked. But what if your partner or someone else close to you raises additional questions that you hadn't considered?

It's best to write down your questions and call your doctor's office as soon as possible, with the understanding that you may talk with a nurse or an assistant. You can also ask your pharmacist questions about your medicine. And there are lots of outside resources, such as books and videotapes (for a list of books, see the Resource Guide at the back of this book). Your public library is a good place to look for these. Members of your family are likely to share your concerns and questions, so you might invite them to join you in gathering information.

If you still have questions, call the office again and ask to speak with the doctor directly.

WHEN DO YOU NEED A MENTAL HEALTH SPECIALIST?

You and your doctor may decide that you should see someone who specializes in working with people who are depressed. Psychiatrists, psychologists, and social workers are mental health specialists trained to deal with depression. Through counseling, these individuals provide a supportive environment for learning better ways of dealing with people and coping with stress and harmful habits. Psychiatrists are also experts on antidepressant medication.

Your doctor may suggest seeing a mental health professional, especially if your depression has not improved after 2 or 3 months of antidepressant therapy, or if you need help with specific problems in your life, such as your marriage or a family crisis. It's a good idea for your mental health specialist to communicate with your doctor about your progress, but he or she can't do so without your approval.

CHAPTER 5

What You Should Know About Antidepressants

After my divorce my doctor prescribed an antidepressant to help with my sleep problems, headaches, low energy, and depression. She said that this antidepressant medication would probably help and that it usually didn't have many side effects. But right away I felt sick to my stomach and jittery. I called my doctor because even though I felt lousy, I knew I shouldn't stop suddenly. She said that nausea and jitteriness can be side effects, but that most likely they would go away. I decided to stick it out a little longer. Over the next week both the nausea and jittery feelings disappeared. I began to feel more energetic and less tired. By the third week I was much less anxious, and my sleep and my mood were a whole lot better. I am really glad I stuck it out.

HOW ANTIDEPRESSANTS WORK

The internal balance of several natural chemicals in our brains influences how we feel emotionally and physically (Figures 5-1 and 5-2). Stress and physical illness can upset this balance. Disturbances in your brain's chemistry can lead to the symptoms of depression: sleep and appetite problems, loss of energy, difficulty concentrating, and increased sensitivity to pain.

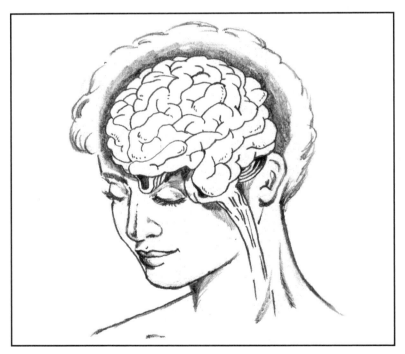

Figure 5-1 — Clinical depression is more than just "the blues" or a "negative attitude." It is associated with changes in the brain's chemical balance.

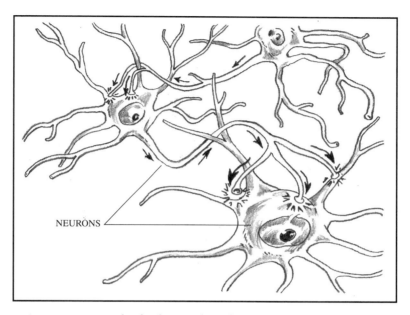

NEURONS

Figure 5-2 — Inside the brain, thoughts, feelings, language, and movement are communicated through a massive network of nerve cells called *neurons*. Electrical impulses carry messages from the beginning of each neuron to its end.

Prescription antidepressant medications reverse that process by replenishing depleted chemical messengers in the brain. These messengers, called *neurotransmitters*, literally carry chemical "messages" between nerve cells in your brain (Figures 5-3, 5-4, 5-5, and 5-6). Two of these neurotransmitters are serotonin and norepinephrine, which have been found to affect mood. The brain needs to receive adequate amounts of these chemicals in order to experience pleasurable sensations. In depression, something goes

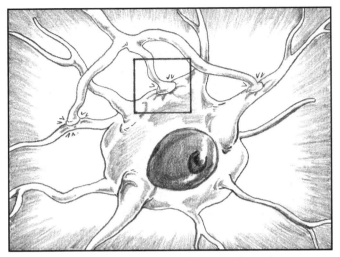

Figure 5-3 — The neurons end in tiny feet that sit on the surface of the adjacent cell.

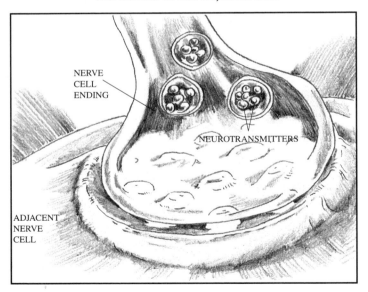

NERVE
CELL
ENDING

NEUROTRANSMITTERS

ADJACENT
NERVE
CELL

Figure 5-4 — These feet contain pouches of chemicals called *neurotransmitters*.

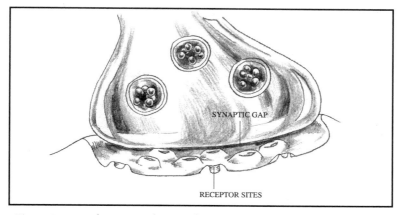

Figure 5-5 — The area where adjacent nerve cells meet is called a *synapse*. A small space called the *synaptic gap* separates the two cells. The neurotransmitters carry the message across the gap to receptor cites on the adjacent cell.

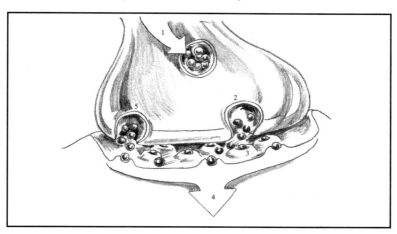

Figure 5-6 — When the electrical signal reaches the end of the cell (1), it triggers the release of neurotransmitters into the gap (2). Normally, the neurotransmitters cross the gap and dock at receptors on the adjacent cell (3), thus continuing the signal (4). The neurotransmitters are then taken back up by the cell they came from (5), a process called *reuptake*.

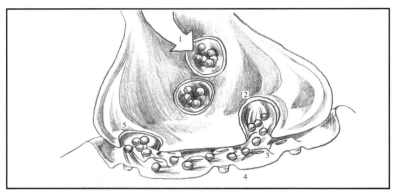

Figure 5-7 — In depression, this communication system between the nerve cells can malfunction. The electrical signal (1) may trigger fewer neurotransmitters to carry the message (2), or they may fail to dock at their receptors (3). As a result, there is no signal to continue on to the adjacent cell (4), and the neurotransmitters may return to the cell that released them (5) without having delivered the message.

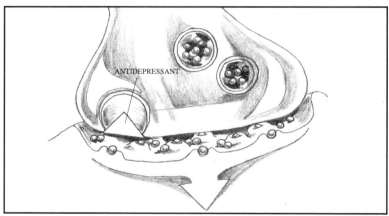

Figure 5-8 — Getting treatment is one way to restore the brain's chemical balance. One treatment—antidepressant drugs— blocks reuptake, giving the neurotransmitters more time to dock at their receptor sites and get their message through to adjacent cells.

wrong, and the serotonin or norepinephrine messengers retreat before they can deliver their message (Figure 5-7).

Newer antidepressant medications, called *serotonin reuptake inhibitors*, or SRIs, prevent the serotonin from retreating too quickly. In effect, they coax serotonin into hanging around long enough to deliver its chemical message (Figure 5-8).

In addition to SRIs, other classes of antidepressants are *tricyclics* and *monoamine oxidase inhibitors*, or MAO inhibitors. *A listing of specific antidepressants in each of these three classes can be found in the Appendix, "A Primer on Antidepressants," at the back of this book.*

WHEN IS AN ANTIDEPRESSANT NECESSARY?

Physicians often describe antidepressants for

- Depression, sadness, or irritability
- Sleep or appetite problems
- Fatigue
- Difficulty with concentration or memory
- Loss of interest in activities that once brought pleasure
- Chronic pain
- Anxiety attacks
- Nervousness or tension

Depression can go away on its own, but taking an antidepressant usually speeds up the recovery process considerably. With no treatment, a depressive episode typically lasts 6–9 months. With medication, however, most people start feeling better in 2–4 weeks.

Some people take antidepressants for only a few months. Others, especially those who tend to develop persistent or recurrent depression, may keep taking them indefinitely, even during periods when they are feeling good. You may hear this referred to as "maintenance" therapy.

FACTS ABOUT ANTIDEPRESSANTS

Antidepressants Are Not Habit Forming

Some people worry about becoming psychologically or physically dependent on antidepressants. Antidepressants are not tranquilizers, and they are NOT habit forming. They increase the supply of chemicals in the brain slowly. For most people, it usually takes 2–4 weeks for the effects of an antidepressant to be felt.

Using Antidepressants Is Not a Sign of Weakness

Is it all right to take an antibiotic to get rid of an infection? Of course it is. If you are prone to depletion of the chemical messengers that keep you feeling good, then taking an antidepressant is just like taking any other effective medicine when you are sick.

It can be hard to make changes in your life when you are depressed. Antidepressants can make those changes easier by increasing your energy, improving your sleep, and helping you concentrate.

Antidepressants Won't Change Your Basic Personality

Antidepressants dramatically change the way some people feel. Others find that the changes are gradual. When the improvement is substantial—if you feel hopeful and energetic for the first time in years, for example—it may seem as if your entire outlook on life has changed. But this is not a change in basic personality. Instead, by correcting an imbalance in brain chemicals, antidepressants allow people to begin to realize their full potential.

Antidepressants Work for Many Different Depressions

Antidepressants relieve the symptoms of depression (such as sadness, tiredness, loss of motivation) regardless of the exact cause. Whether you will benefit from antidepressants depends on how severe your depression is and how long it lasts, not on why it started.

SIDE EFFECTS

Most people who take antidepressants experience some side effects, at least for a little while. Side effects may be annoying, but they are rarely dangerous to your health and are usually manageable. Tell your doctor about any side effects you are experiencing. Working together, the two of you can find the right antidepressant and the right dosage for you.

Use the Appendix, "A Primer on Antidepressants," to familiarize yourself with the different classes of antidepressants available. Your doctor may suggest one or a combination of these drugs. This appendix will give you an idea of some of the side effects you can expect, but as always, it is best to ask your doctor or pharmacist for a more detailed description of possible side effects before taking any medication.

How to Manage Side Effects

Side effects usually occur in the first 2 weeks of beginning an antidepressant, and then gradually ease as your body adapts to the medicine. Because it may take as long as 4 weeks for the antidepressant to start working, some patients feel a little worse before they begin to feel better and may give up on the medication too soon.

If you are bothered by side effects, discuss them with your doctor. DO NOT stop taking the medicine on your own. Your doctor can help you determine if you're experiencing a minor side effect that will go away soon, or if you need to switch to a different antidepressant. It's common for doctors to adjust the dosage or to switch medications. Your goal is to get the best possible therapeutic effect while keeping side effects to a minimum.

Chris's story:

When I first started the antidepressant, I had problems with dry mouth and constipation. My doctor said that these could be side effects and that they would probably ease over time. He suggested that I drink more fluids, exercise regularly, and add fiber to my diet. Over the next 2 or 3 weeks these side effects did ease.

Sharon's story:

My doctor advised me to stay on my antidepressant a good 6 months even after I was better so that my depression wouldn't come back. But over the next 3 months I started to crave sweets and the next thing I knew I had put on 15 pounds! At my next appointment I told my doctor about my craving for sweets and gaining weight. He said it could be because I was taking a tricyclic antidepressant and suggested that I switch to one of the new antidepressants that don't usually have this side effect.

FINDING AN ANTIDEPRESSANT THAT WORKS FOR YOU

All antidepressants work well. But not all of them work well for everybody. Approximately 7 out of 10 people respond to the first or second antidepressant they try. By working together, you and your doctor will be able to figure out if the antidepressant you start with is the right one for you. If you try more than one and still can't tolerate the side effects or you just don't feel any better, your doctor may want to consult with a psychiatrist or refer you to a mental health specialist.

CHAPTER 6

What You Should Know About Psychotherapy

My doctor suggested that I start seeing a therapist. She must think I'm really bad off. I've heard about those therapists who never say anything and keep you coming back for years. How is that supposed to help?

WHAT IS PSYCHOTHERAPY?

It is possible that your doctor will recommend you see a psychotherapist for help in dealing with your depression. Psychotherapy involves talking about problems with a therapist and developing strategies to deal with them. Psychologists, psychiatrists, and licensed clinical social workers can provide this type of care.

Psychotherapy can help you get more pleasure and satisfaction out of life. It can make you more aware of your feelings and thoughts and the ways your actions affect others. It can teach you new things about yourself. It permits you to try out new ways of thinking, behaving, and interacting with others in an atmosphere of support and encouragement.

Therapy can also help you change the way you deal with problems in your life. Therapy won't make those problems disappear, of course. It won't make a lousy job better or entirely take away the pain of losing a loved one. But therapy can help you learn better ways of handling the issues of everyday living.

TYPES OF THERAPISTS AND THERAPY

Several different types of mental health professionals can provide psychotherapy. Psychiatrists are medical doctors (MDs) who can prescribe medications as well as provide psychotherapy. Most other psychotherapists do not write prescriptions. These include psychologists (who may have either a PhD or a master's degree), social workers (who have a master's degree in social work), counselors with a master's degree, and mental health nurses, who are registered nurses (RNs). Practitioners who are not MDs often work with physicians when they think prescription medications might complement psychotherapy.

Across all these professional groups, you're likely to find a wide variety in the kinds of psychotherapy that individual therapists practice. The five most common kinds of therapy are

1. Interpersonal therapy
2. Cognitive-behavioral therapy
3. Behavioral therapy
4. Problem-solving therapy (PST)
5. Psychodynamic (or family-of-origin) therapy

You might find that a particular psychotherapist offers only behavioral therapy, whereas another may prefer a psychodynamic approach. But all therapists are trained to provide support, encouragement, and education and should be able to help you create worthwhile changes in your life.

Four of the five main types of psychotherapy for depression have been evaluated extensively: interpersonal therapy, cognitive-behavioral therapy, behavioral therapy, and problem-solving therapy. For people with mild to moderate depression, all four have been found to be as effective as antidepressants in reducing the symptoms of depression. For severe depression, antidepressant medications are more effective than psychotherapy.

Psychotherapy takes a little longer than medication to begin showing results, but after 3 or 4 months psychotherapy and antidepressants appear to work equally well. Some patients benefit from a combination of antidepressant and psychotherapy. Antidepressants can help relieve many of the physical and emotional symptoms of depression, restoring the energy and emotional reserves that can help you benefit from psychotherapy.

Therapy may be done on a one-on-one basis, through couples counseling, or in a group setting. Choose one that bests suits your personality and your needs.

In addition to being good listeners, therapists act as educators and coaches for their patients. For most people, therapy begins to alleviate depression in a month or two.

Interpersonal Therapy

Personal crises such as a death in the family, a divorce, or marital or family difficulties are often the trigger for an episode of depression. Because problems in close relationships are among the most common risks for depression, interpersonal therapy was developed to treat people whose depression is triggered by these problems.

Many people who seek interpersonal therapy have trouble grieving for the loss of a loved one or taking on new roles, or they find themselves in conflicts with loved ones. They may also lack the social skills that make it possible to have warm and satisfying relationships with others. Interpersonal therapy is based on principles of more traditional (or psychodynamic) psychotherapy. One important principle is that our difficulties in current relationships are often related to beliefs or assumptions about ourselves and others. Relationships in early life may be important influences on those beliefs and assumptions.

A typical interpersonal therapy session will concentrate on your current problems and relationships. The therapist may help you understand your thoughts and emotions after divorce or the arrival of a new baby, for example. Or the therapist may encourage you to talk about the pain of losing a loved one.

Cognitive-Behavioral Therapy

One of the assumptions underlying cognitive-behavioral therapy is that stress can lead to a repetitive cycle of negative thought patterns and that these thought patterns then cause depressive moods.

When criticized by a supervisor, a person who is not vulnerable to depression might react by thinking, "I'll have to improve this aspect of my work," or "The boss must be having a bad day." In a person with a tendency toward depression, however, the same criticism can trigger a host of negative thoughts that turn into beliefs about the person's overall competence and self-worth. A supervisor's comment about a missed deadline might lead to conclusions like, "See, I'm failing again," or "This just shows how incompetent I am as a worker and provider for my family."

We all have thoughts like this occasionally, but in people with depression such thought patterns are more persistent and are triggered more easily.

Cognitive-behavioral therapists can help by

- Identifying these recurrent negative thought patterns
- Encouraging you to challenge negative thought patterns
- Gradually helping you to replace the negative patterns with positive thoughts

In a typical session, you and your therapist may review a weekly "homework" assignment. For example, you might be asked to keep track of your moods and activities every day. If depressed feelings begin, you will be able to backtrack and identify the precipitating stress or event and describe the negative thoughts that event triggered. In this way you may discover that a certain event (such as criticism by the boss) did not cause depression, but certain negative thought patterns on your part led to a decline in mood after the event.

The therapist functions as a teacher and coach, often leading you through a logical line of questioning such as "What's the worse thing that would happen if you did that?" This would be followed by "And then what would happen?"

Behavioral Therapy

When you are depressed, you stop doing things that reward you with a sense of pleasure or accomplishment. To counter this, behavioral therapy helps you plan and carry out activities that are enjoyable and rewarding.

Behavioral therapy also helps you improve your ability to solve problems and communicate with others, which enables you to become more active and effective at work and at home. The result: both your mood and your self-esteem improve.

Behavioral therapists encourage you especially to increase the amount of rewarding social activities in your life. The love and support of friends and family can be a big help in challenging negative thought patterns. Training in relaxation and in problem-solving may also be part of behavioral therapy.

Behavioral therapy is very action oriented. As in cognitive therapy, you should expect to have homework assignments—for example, you may be encouraged to structure at least one positive activity into each day, such as taking a walk with a friend or going out to dinner with your spouse. In a typical session, you and your therapist might review the previous week's homework to evaluate its effect on your mood.

Problem-Solving Therapy (PST)

This type of therapy focuses on improving your problem-solving skills. Major life problems (like financial difficulties or conflicts at work) are also common triggers for depression. Depression in turn interferes with your ability to manage life problems effectively—even minor stresses can leave you feeling overwhelmed. This self-reinforcing cycle is another part of the downward spiral of depression.

Problem-solving therapy is designed to improve your skills for managing major and minor life problems. The idea is to follow a series of specific steps:

1. Breaking a big problem into a number of smaller (and more manageable) pieces
2. Identifying a wide range of possible solutions
3. Choosing one possible solution to try first—and trying it
4. Evaluating the results of your experiment and (if necessary) making any changes in your plan

In a typical session, you and your therapist would begin by identifying a problem to work on. It's important to start with a problem that will allow some progress. During that session (or a series of sessions), you'd follow the steps listed above and evaluate your progress. The goal is to develop your skills and confidence in applying these steps to other problems (large and small) outside the therapy sessions.

Psychodynamic Therapy

A fifth type of therapy, known as psychodynamic (or family-of-origin) therapy, can help relieve depressive symptoms in some people. This therapy focuses on helping you understand how past family experiences affect your current ways of thinking and acting. Psychodynamic therapy can be provided on an individual basis, through couples counseling, or in a group therapy setting.

Sessions are likely to deal with early experiences that may have affected self-image or self-esteem. Some therapists encourage you to talk about your dreams, which may be useful in revealing unconscious motivations or desires. The therapist may ask questions and point out patterns of behavior. Generally there's little if any "homework" of the sort that's commonly associated with cognitive-behavioral and behavioral therapies.

Many people find that psychodynamic therapy helps them develop insight into their problems, but the evidence for its effectiveness in depression is not as strong as it is for interpersonal, cognitive-behavioral, behavioral, or problem-solving therapy. Psychodynamic therapy tends to focus on long-term changes in ways of coping with stress and relationships and less on immediate relief of symptoms.

HOW DO I FIND A THERAPIST?

You can get names and other information about psychotherapists from your doctor, friends, or family members. Most university departments of psychiatry or psychology can give you referrals as well. State psychological associations and the National Depressive and Manic-Depressive Association also operate referral networks. Other groups, such as women's therapy referral networks or crisis centers, also may be able to provide you with names and phone numbers. You'll find additional sources listed in the Resource Guide at the back of this book.

What Can I Expect During the First Few Sessions?

During the first visit, your therapist will probably want to complete a thorough assessment of your depression. He or she is likely to ask you about your current difficulties and any related problems in the past, about your medical history, and about your use of alcohol and other drugs. The therapist should also ask if others in your family have a history of depression or other mental disorders. He or she may also ask permission to talk to your medical doctor in order to rule out other possible causes of depression, such as physical illness or the side effects of medications.

During your first few visits, plan on working with your therapist to formulate a design for your therapy, and set realistic goals for your progress. If you are working within the guidelines of a health insurance plan, you may be forced to restrict your goals to what you can reasonably expect to accomplish in a limited time. In order to continue therapy beyond what insurance will cover, you may be able to negotiate a reasonable fee with your therapist.

Before starting therapy, ask what the treatment is likely to cost. If it's more than you can afford, don't be ashamed to say so. The therapist may be able to work with you to control costs. For example, you may be able to see the therapist once every 2 weeks rather than every week.

In the first couple of sessions, make sure you feel comfortable with your therapist. For therapy to be successful, you should feel that you can trust your therapist and that he or she is attentive and understanding. A strong, trusting alliance with the therapist is the best predictor of success in therapy. You may not always be comfortable when you are asked to try new behaviors or confront difficult issues, but overall you should feel that your therapist is on your side.

HOW DO I KNOW IF IT'S WORKING?

You are the best judge! After about 6 weeks of psychotherapy, you should notice some improvement. If by 8 to 10 weeks you are not feeling much better, consider switching to a different therapist or a different type of treatment. Discuss your concerns with your therapist and/or your doctor. If you haven't been supplementing therapy with antidepressant medication, you might want to talk about this option with your doctor.

CHAPTER 7

When Is Treatment Finished?

After my third relapse, I agreed with my doctor that I should stay on antidepressants indefinitely. My depression is so painful and disruptive to my life that I want to do anything I can to try to prevent a recurrence.

Most people with depression do get better after several months, or even sooner with effective treatment. If you're like most people, you may feel tempted to stop treatment as soon as you feel better. You're almost certainly better off taking some time to consider what length of treatment is most reasonable for you. This chapter includes some specific information you should consider.

WHAT'S THE MINIMUM LENGTH OF TREATMENT?

While antidepressant medications may have significant positive effects in only 2 to 3 weeks, most doctors consider 5 or 6 months to be a minimum effective treatment. You may be tempted to stop taking medication once you're feeling better, but the risk of slipping back into depression is quite high for at least a few months. Most studies of psychotherapy for depression also consider at least 4 months of treatment to be an effective "dose." For these reasons, we cannot recommend that anyone discontinue depression treatment after only a month or two. If you feel you really cannot continue longer, you should discuss with your doctor or therapist whether a different treatment (rather than stopping treatment) might be appropriate. For some people, longer-term treatment is clearly indicated. Whether you should consider longer-term treatment depends on your risk of a return to depression (or a relapse).

WHO NEEDS MORE THAN THE MINIMUM?

Each of us is different, but your personal risk is somewhat predictable. As in many other situations, the best predictor of the future is the past. The more episodes of depression you have had, the more severe they have been and the longer they have lasted, the more likely your depression will recur. The risk of recurrence is also related to what goes on in your daily life. New, stressful events and long-term difficulties can trigger a relapse into depression. You should consider longer-term treatment if you have had more chronic depression (for example, depression lasting longer than 2 years) or more frequent recurrences (for example, at least three episodes of depression in the past 5 years).

THE EVIDENCE FOR MAINTENANCE MEDICATION

Long-term or maintenance use of antidepressants is one way to prevent a relapse or recurrence of depression. We have strong evidence that longer-term use of medications reduces the risk of relapse for people who have had frequent recurrences of depression. In one study, only one out of five people who continued taking the same dose of antidepressant became depressed again within 2 years, compared with four out of five of those who took a placebo or dummy pill. Because of these findings, many doctors now recommend long-term, continuous use of antidepressants for people who have had three or more episodes of depression, or who have had chronic depression lasting 2 or more years. These same studies also show that long-term use of antidepressants is quite safe.

Even after you've been on medication for several months, you may still experience some side effects. Some problems that seemed tolerable when your antidepressant was lifting you out of depression (like dry mouth or constipation) may bother you more as time goes by and you feel better. Other side effects (like sexual problems or weight gain) may only become obvious after a few months. If side effects are a problem (and certainly if you're thinking about stopping your antidepressant because of them), discuss them with your doctor. Adjusting the dosage or changing to a different antidepressant often helps.

If you decide to continue taking your antidepressant, try not to rethink your decision every day. Even if your antidepressant is working just as it should, you'll still have better days and worse ones. Because antidepressants work slowly, day-to-day fluctuations in your mood probably don't say much about how well your antidepressant works or whether it's necessary. Second, frequently rethinking your decision about antidepressants can waste a lot of energy. It's best to "reenlist" for some set period of time, like 6 months or a year. When the time is up, you can discuss your situation with your doctor and decide whether to reenlist again.

FIVE BAD REASONS FOR STOPPING
ANTIDEPRESSANT MEDICATION

The section above presents the rational, scientific evidence about continuing or discontinuing antidepressant medications. Most of us, however, have a sizable dose of the irrational in many of our decisions—including decisions about medical treatment. You are less likely to be influenced by these "less than rational" reasons if you recognize them for what they are. Here's a list of some "less than rational" (but very common) reasons why people stop taking antidepressant medication:

1. I couldn't pick up the refill before the holiday weekend, and I've been doing OK for two days now.
2. I've moved, and I can't stand having to tell my whole story to a new doctor.
3. I wouldn't want my new girlfriend to know I've been taking this medication.
4. My family keeps telling me I'm sick; stopping my medication will prove that I'm really just fine.
5. I had to change health plans, and it is too much hassle to get a referral to a new doctor.

THE EVIDENCE FOR MAINTENANCE PSYCHOTHERAPY

The evidence for the effectiveness of long-term or maintenance psychotherapy in preventing relapse of depression is not as strong as the evidence for maintenance medication. Some recent studies have suggested that cognitive-behavioral therapy may significantly decrease the risk of relapse. Other studies suggest that continuing regular (but less frequent) psychotherapy sessions after you feel better may reduce the risk of relapse. Continuing psychotherapy may, however, be helpful for specific individuals. You and your therapist should discuss your individual situation to determine what's best for you.

CONTINUING GOOD SELF-CARE IS NOT OPTIONAL

As the information in this chapter suggests, maintenance or long-term treatment (with either antidepressant medications or psychotherapy) is a personal decision. Some people will discontinue treatment after 6 months and continue to do well. Others will decide to continue for much longer. You and your doctor should consider your individual situation before deciding what is most appropriate for you.

In contrast, continuing to practice good self-care is always a good idea. Regardless of your past experience with depression or your experience with depression treatment, you'll reduce your future risk of depression by maintaining your self-care skills. Chapter 24 of this book, "Maintaining Gains and Preventing Relapse," will help you to create a written plan to continue practicing good self-care. If you haven't yet read Chapter 24 (or if you've read it but didn't write down your plan), you may want to do so now.

CHAPTER 8

What Family and Friends Should Know

This chapter is for your friends and family. It may answer some of their questions and help clear up misunderstandings about depression. You may want to share this section with the people in your life whom you feel comfortable talking to about your depression.

IS THIS MY FAULT?

Because the causes of depression often are not clear, it's easy for family members or close friends to feel guilty about their loved one's illness. Instead of worrying about what you may have done in the past, try to focus on specific things you can do from now on. Help to create a fresh start that will focus on prospects for a brighter future. Someone who is depressed will frequently be irritable or show less interest in your relationship. Don't take it personally.

WHAT IF I JUST MAKE THINGS WORSE?

Self-blame is a big part of depression; try not to fall into that trap yourself. You won't always know the right thing to say, but don't let that stop you from talking. It's more important that you let your loved one know you care and that you are available to help. Persistence and good intentions will go a long way.

WHAT SHOULD I KNOW ABOUT ANTIDEPRESSANTS?

A doctor's recommendation to use antidepressant medication often raises questions or concerns. If your friend or family member has started using an antidepressant (or is trying to decide whether to begin one), you probably have several questions. You can be most helpful to your friend or family member by:

- Having an open discussion about the pros and cons of antidepressant treatment. You can be a valuable sounding board, but the depressed person must make his or her own decision.

- Trying to support the decision if your friend or family member decides to take an antidepressant. Most people beginning antidepressant treatment do enough second-guessing all by themselves.
- Agreeing in advance how you'll handle the day-to-day medicine schedule. Some people appreciate reminders, while others see reminders as nagging. Decide together how you will handle it.
- Trying not to make medication a moral issue. Taking an antidepressant is about restoring health, not about being weak. Stopping antidepressants too early is a far more common problem than staying on them too long. Avoid questions like "Do you still need to take those pills?"

WHAT SHOULD I AVOID DOING OR SAYING?

Even if you mean well and try hard, there may still be difficult times. Here are some common "don'ts" to keep in mind:

- **Don't say, "Can't you just get a grip on yourself!"** Depression is not laziness, but sometimes you may feel that way. If your depressed friend or family member can't do the things he or she normally does, you may feel burdened and even irritated. It helps to remember the times when you felt especially down, frustrated, or discouraged yourself.

- **Don't use the silent treatment.** Sometimes you may say nothing for fear of saying something wrong. Silence can leave lots of room for a depressed person's negative or self-critical interpretations. When there's room for doubt, people who feel depressed tend to blame themselves. If you don't know what to say or do, try asking. Or just tell the truth: "I'd like to help, but I don't know what to say."

- **Don't say, "You're acting like you didn't take that pill today."** Disagreements and upsetting times are a part of everyday life and usually won't have anything to do with whether or not someone took an antidepressant on a particular day. It may be a good idea to help someone you care for remember to take medicine on schedule, but don't bring it up in the middle of an argument. Try not to associate taking antidepressant medication with negative events.

HOW CAN I HELP?

Encourage Regular Activity

Physical and social activity are effective natural antidepressants. Depression drains away energy and motivation, so depressed people often withdraw from enjoyable activities. The way to reverse that feeling is regular activities that bring them pleasure or build their confidence.

You can help by being a partner. Try to schedule something rewarding every day (for example, physical activity, entertainment or social activities). Set a specific time and don't take "no" for an answer. Start slowly, but keep a steady pace. Offer lots of encouragement, and take it easy on the criticism.

Help Turn Mountains Back Into Molehills

To someone who feels depressed, every road looks like a steep uphill climb. Daily problems seem so overwhelming that it's hard to get started on any solutions. Even a little bit of help from you can help shrink some of those problems down to a manageable size.

Here are some simple steps to follow:

- Break a large problem down into small pieces
- Decide which part of the problem to take on first
- Identify one or two small steps to start with
- Set a specific time and place to get started

Reminisce About Good Times

People who are depressed find it hard to remember that life has ever been anything but bleak. Memories of past successes, accomplishments and good times are poisoned by how bad things seem right now. You can help by holding on to a more optimistic view of the past. Don't argue; just offer a few gentle reminders like, "You were better at that than you remember." People with depression are very critical of themselves, so support and nonjudgmental love of family and friends are especially important.

Get Involved In Depression Treatment

Part of depression is feeling terribly alone. Offer to help in any way that seems appropriate to you. For example, the two of you could do some reading about depression and talk about it together. Or you might go along on visits to a doctor or counselor.

Sometimes problems in a relationship can contribute to depression, or depression can cause serious problems in a relationship. If relationship difficulties are a major source of stress, joint counseling can be helpful.

Let The Depressed Person Know When You See Improvement

You may notice improvements in mood, attitude and behavior before the depressed person does. Tell him or her if you see improvement, especially if treatment seems to be working.

HOW CAN I HELP KEEP DEPRESSION FROM COMING BACK?

Most depressed people feel significantly better after 1 or 2 months of treatment. Unfortunately, depression sometimes returns especially if treatment such as antidepressant medication is stopped too early.

Once things are better, you can help by watching out for early warning-signs. If depression starts to creep back into someone's life, friends or family may be the first to notice. You may spot clues like sleep problems, irritability or withdrawal from social situations.

When things are going well, it might be a good idea to sit down together to make a list of early warning signs or clues that depression is resuming. Talk about a schedule for regular self-evaluations like those we describe in Chapter 24, "Maintaining Gains and Preventing Relapse." It's best to agree in advance about how you can bring up your concerns in the most helpful way. If you've worked out a plan in advance, you'll be able to mention warning signs of depression without seeming critical.

CHAPTER 9

Plain Talk About Suicide

WHO IS AT RISK?

Feelings of discouragement or even hopelessness are a common part of depression. As many as 30% of people with major depression will have thoughts of suicide at some point. Although these thoughts are always a cause of concern, most people who have suicidal thoughts never act on them. Among those who suffer from depression, suicide is more common among men, those over age 50, and those with significant medical problems.

GETTING THROUGH A CRISIS

Thoughts of death or suicide are a common sign of depression. Urges or plans to act on suicidal thoughts are a sign that immediate attention is necessary. When you are in such a crisis, it can be hard to think of much else. The following steps may be useful if you are having suicidal thoughts.

Talk About It

An honest discussion with friends, family, and your doctor or therapist is the best way to resist suicidal thoughts. Talking about suicidal thoughts doesn't increase the danger. Many times, an open discussion about suicidal thoughts and feelings of hopelessness is the first step toward recovery. In most cities or counties, telephone crisis counselors are available 24 hours a day to offer support and referrals for emergency treatment. Look in the Yellow Pages or call information for a hotline in your area.

Make a Plan for Getting Through

Discuss with your doctor, friends, or family exactly how you'll be able to get through the next few days. Schedule activities that will keep you involved with family, friends, or coworkers, even if it is just a minor activity like taking a walk. Don't be shy about asking family or friends to spend some time with you. Write out your plan on how you will spend the next few days—the more specific, the better—and keep it where you are sure to see it frequently. Sometimes, knowing that you have a schedule to stick to can give you the boost that you need to get through a tough time.

Avoid Alcohol and Drugs

Suicidal thoughts and alcohol are an especially dangerous combination. Not only can alcohol or drugs worsen feelings of depression, they increase the chance you might act impulsively. If you are taking an antidepressant, you should be avoiding alcohol anyway. Alcohol is a depressant, and it can counteract the effects that the medication is trying to achieve.

Don't Let Depression Cloud Your Thinking

When you are depressed, everything looks worse than it really is. You may feel that others would be better off without you, even though they tell you that isn't so. Or you may get bogged down in a mental debate over whether life is worthwhile. Don't let the negative thoughts win out. When you start feeling this way, try to clear your mind by going to a movie, taking a walk or calling a friend.

PREVENTIVE MEDICINE

Even if you don't feel urges to act on suicidal thoughts, *thinking of suicide* is a sign of trouble. If you find yourself thinking frequently about death or suicide, consider the following steps:

- **Get treatment.** The most effective prevention of suicide is effective treatment of depression. If you have thoughts about suicide, you should certainly consult your doctor. If you continue to have suicidal thoughts despite treatment, be sure to tell your doctor or therapist. A change in treatment may be necessary.

- **Structure your time.** Long periods of time alone or unoccupied can give depression the opportunity to take control. Feelings of hopelessness or suicide can seem much more reasonable when you are alone than when you are busy or spending time with family or friends.

CAN ANTIDEPRESSANT MEDICATIONS CAUSE SUICIDE?

Reports of a few isolated cases have suggested the possibility that antidepressant medication may create or worsen suicidal ideas. Even though these reports have received extensive media coverage, the best scientific evidence suggests otherwise.

Antidepressant medications can reduce suicidal thoughts and suicide attempts. Although it is possible that some people may have unusual or extreme reactions to certain medications, concern about suicide is an argument *for* antidepressant treatment, not against it.

CHAPTER 10

Depression and Your Body

When the doctor first said "multiple sclerosis," I felt so pan-
icked that I really didn't hear anything else she said that
day. It felt like the end of the world. It wasn't, but my world
is different and it's taken some work to adjust to it. I can't
always do the things I used to, and I have to adjust my
expectations. Sometimes the medications make me feel foggy
and worn out, and I've certainly had some low times. Try-
ing to stay active and finding support from other people
with MS have helped keep me from getting too discouraged.

Your body and your mind are more than just close
neighbors. They're two aspects of the same whole. Physical changes in your body (caused my medical problems,
medications, aging, etc.) can have big effects on your
mood. Your thoughts and feelings also have significant

THE DEPRESSION HELPBOOK

effects on how you take care of yourself as well as how you feel and interpret what's happening in your body. This chapter describes some of the ways that your mind and your body interact with each other—and how you can make that interaction a positive one.

MEDICAL CONDITIONS AND DEPRESSION

Chronic medical problems, such as diabetes or heart disease, can be major sources of physical discomfort and psychological stress. Many people with chronic medical illnesses experience some level of fatigue, discouragement, and depression. Some medical problems may have a specific biologic effect on your mood. Certain neurological conditions, such as stroke, multiple sclerosis, Parkinson's disease, and traumatic head injuries, can disrupt the brain's normal chemical balance. Other diseases that can affect mood include endocrine or hormone disorders like hypothyroidism. Chapter 11 includes more information about the relationship between medical illness and depression and about how you can manage that combination more effectively.

For women, hormonal changes during the menstrual cycle, or at menopause, can have significant effects on mood. Depression after childbirth is especially common, and sometimes serious. Chapter 12 includes more information about depression and women's health.

Prescription medications can also have a negative effect on mood. Commonly prescribed medications that may contribute to depression include certain blood pressure medicines, birth control pills, hormone replacement therapy, and steroid medications. Sleeping pills and tranquilizers, when taken for long periods, also can contribute to depression.

Some medications have side effects that become more pronounced with age. If depression is one of these side effects, then an older person is more likely to become depressed when taking the medication than a younger person. If you are concerned that a medication you are taking for a chronic condition may be affecting your mood, be sure to mention it to your doctor.

ANXIETY AND DEPRESSION

Most people with depression also suffer anxiety problems. Anxiety is associated with depletion of the same brain chemicals that are reduced in depression.

Symptoms of anxiety include feeling keyed up and nervous, difficulty tuning out worries, and muscle tension. Intense anxiety or panic attack is characterized by pounding heart, tight and painful chest, shortness of breath, sweating, shakiness, light-headedness, sensations of heat or cold, or a sense that something disastrous is happening.

Anxiety attacks may make people fear places where there are crowds or where leaving will be difficult or embarrassing. Anxiety or panic attacks also cause some people to think that something is physically wrong, because severe symptoms that can accompany an attack, like chest pain or shortness of breath, make them think they are having a heart attack or stroke.

If you find yourself avoiding situations because they make you afraid or anxious, it's even more important to stay active and involved. Avoidance actually increases anxiety. Confronting your fears will give power back to you, and it will help you feel more in control.

Fortunately, many of the same treatments that work for depression also work for the anxiety associated with depression.

PAIN AND DEPRESSION

Pain can contribute to depression in a number of ways. Chronic headaches, backaches, diabetic neuropathy, abdominal pain, or other discomfort can get you down and keep you from enjoying life. Pain can upset normal sleep patterns and cause decreased energy. Pain can also limit your activities, causing you to withdraw from social situations that you would normally enjoy. This sense of isolation and of missing out on the fun side of life can bring on depression.

When you are in pain, it is sometimes difficult to see anything in a positive light. But if you suffer from physical pain and depression, finding ways of managing that pain will be an important part of your treatment plan. Staying as active as possible—both physically and socially—is crucial, but if your pain is severe, your doctor may also prescribe pain medication.

Increased Sensitivity to Pain

Pain messages are electrical impulses that travel to your brain along nerve fibers. When you're depressed, this finely tuned electrical system may work too well. Depression can amplify pain signals, just as if you turned up the volume on your stereo. Fortunately, these pain sensations can also be dampened or turned down.

This does not mean that your pain is imaginary or in any sense not "real." But there are things you can do to feel less pain.

Recurrent or Chronic Pain

Completely eliminating pain may not be a realistic goal, but improving the quality of your life certainly is. Here are some suggestions for dealing with chronic pain:

- **Stay as active as you can.** Withdrawing from social and physical activities can focus more of your attention on your pain. For many kinds of pain, physical activity is actually helpful, not harmful. Physical exercise raises levels of *endorphins*, the body's natural painkillers.

- **Put some static into the system.** Other physical sensations interfere with pain perception, and you can take advantage of that. Sending another kind of signal down the same path can shut off the flow of pain messages. Some examples: massage, hot or cold compresses, and acupuncture.

- **Learn to refocus your attention.** Pain is hard to ignore; that's how your brain was designed. Learning to redirect your attention away from pain messages takes practice, but it can help. You may want to try some of the relaxation techniques mentioned later on in this book.

ABOUT PRESCRIPTION PAIN MEDICATIONS

Prescription pain medications can decrease the intensity of pain signals. Unfortunately, they can also introduce a new set of problems. First, regular use of narcotic pain medicines can reduce your energy level, lower your mood, cause constipation, and decrease your motivation. All of these effects can make pain worse. Second, for some people regular use of prescription painkillers can lead to tolerance or psychological dependence. This means that you may need to take more and more of them to get the same effect you did at the beginning, and you are likely to feel much worse when you try to stop taking them.

Most doctors prefer to limit prescription medications to short-term use. Your doctor or other health care provider should supervise more than 2 weeks of regular use. Also, remember that painkillers should be taken on a schedule. If you wait until you're in terrible pain to take the medication, you'll probably need more of it. If you're taking pain pills more than once a day, plan to take them at specific times whether you are in pain or not.

ANTIDEPRESSANTS AND PAIN

Antidepressants can help with pain in two ways. First, antidepressants directly affect your body's pain signals. In fact, many people who are not depressed but who have chronic pain get relief from antidepressants. They help turn down the volume on all kinds of pain sensations so that pain is not as distressing or disabling. Second, antidepressants can increase your energy level and make it easier for you to become active again, which, in turn, helps reduce pain.

Both of these effects build up gradually. This means that antidepressants will be more effective if you take them every day, not just when you are in pain.

CHAPTER 11

Depression and Chronic Medical Illness

The doctor said it was only a "tiny heart attack," but it really set me back. I was afraid to exert myself, and it seemed that everyone treated me like I was just about to keel over. I felt useless, I was worried all the time, and my sex life just disappeared. My doctor kept after me to start exercising, but that just made me feel guilty. Then he suggested a group exercise and rehab program for heart patients. I've never been a health fanatic or much of a "joiner," but getting together for the exercise class has really helped. I realize that I was really afraid of what would happen if I pushed myself, and being with other people gave me a lot more confidence. I feel like I've accomplished something, and I've learned to lighten up and think more about having fun.

THE MIND-BODY CONNECTION IN CHRONIC ILLNESS

How Chronic Illness Affects Your Mood

Some chronic medical illnesses may have direct effects on mood and energy. Thyroid conditions often cause fatigue and low mood. Neurological conditions like stroke or multiple sclerosis may affect parts of the brain that regulate mood and emotions. Major medical events like a heart attack or surgery can increase levels of stress hormones leading to feelings of depression and anxiety.

More often, chronic illness can contribute to depression because of physical discomfort, disturbed sleep, or limitations on your activities. As described in Chapter 2, withdrawing from pleasant or rewarding activities is both a major effect and a major cause of depression. Persistent pain is also a common cause of depression and fatigue.

Depression and Physical Symptoms

Depression is not just a "mental" problem. Some of the most disabling symptoms of depression are physical ones like fatigue, trouble sleeping, or persistent pain. It can be difficult to sort out whether pain or fatigue is caused by depression or medical problems, but that's because they can't really be sorted out. Medical problems and depression often work together to cause physical symptoms. Pain or fatigue from any cause seems much more severe and disabling when you feel discouraged or hopeless.

Biological Effects of Depression

Depression is a mental and physical condition—with significant changes in hormones and chemical messengers throughout your body. Some of these effects are obvious: changes in appetite, fatigue, disturbed sleep. Some other changes don't cause immediate symptoms but can have important effects on your health. Depression affects levels of cortisol and other stress hormones leading to increases in blood sugar and increased risk of heart disease. Effects on blood clotting can increase risk of stroke or heart attack.

Depression and Self-Care

Feeling depressed can also get in the way of taking care of yourself the way you hope to. Managing a chronic illness often involves taking medication regularly and may involve some kind of self-monitoring (like checking your blood sugar on your own). Sticking to those routines can be difficult when you feel that nothing is worth the effort. Chronic illness may make it even more important to make lifestyle changes like stopping smoking, exercising regularly, or losing weight. Those changes can seem nearly impossible when you feel discouraged or depressed.

Does This Mean That the Problem Is All in My Head?

A chronic illness like diabetes or emphysema certainly isn't a figment of your imagination. You didn't make it up, and you certainly can't wish it away. What you can do, however, is take charge as best you can. When your mood is better, any burden is easier to bear. So the problem is certainly not in your head, but the beginning of the solution is.

DEPRESSION AND SPECIFIC CHRONIC ILLNESSES

Diabetes

Nearly one-third of people with diabetes experience some level of depression, ranging from mild to serious. Depression and diabetes are related on several different levels. Depression appears to have a direct effect on control of blood sugar. Depression and stress can lead to hormonal changes that increase blood sugar and reduce the effect of natural insulin. Depression also makes it more difficult to manage diabetes effectively. Taking steps like changing your diet, exercising more, and losing weight are difficult even when you're feeling good and may seem overwhelming when you're depressed. Symptoms of diabetes can also contribute to depression. Changes in blood sugar level may cause fatigue and interfere with your concentration. Eye damage or nerve damage from diabetes may prevent you from doing some of the things you've always enjoyed.

Heart Disease

As many as 25 percent of people with heart disease may also experience depression. Depression is especially common after heart attack or bypass surgery. Some of the relationship between heart disease and depression is biological. Depression may affect stress hormones and blood clotting, leading to increased risk of heart disease. Psychological changes can play a major role as well. Heart disease often changes the way you think about yourself, and you may find yourself withdrawing from people and activities you've enjoyed. You may be fearful that "overdoing it" (even in a positive way) might be dangerous. Feeling depressed also makes it much more difficult to quit smoking or start an exercise program. It's also easy to feel fatalistic or hopeless, thinking that the damage is already done so there's not much point in making changes.

Arthritis

The central symptoms of arthritis are persistent pain and immobility, and it's hard to imagine a more discouraging combination. Chronic or recurrent pain certainly contributes to depression, and feeling depressed makes any pain problem much harder to bear. Pain often interferes with sleep, another important influence on your mood and energy. Limits on your activities can contribute to the vicious cycle of depression: the less you do the worse you feel, and the worse you feel the less you do. For some people, arthritis medications (like prednisone) can also have a big effect on mood.

Stroke

A stroke is a brain injury, so it's not surprising that depression is common after stroke. Sometimes one or more small strokes (too small to cause obvious weakness or numbness in your body) can trigger depression. Major strokes are a devastating event and may severely limit your mobility, communication, and independence. Those major limitations may contribute to the vicious cycle of depression.

GENERAL STRATEGIES FOR MANAGING CHRONIC ILLNESS

Turning Mountains Back into Molehills

When you run into problems that seem impossible to solve, try breaking them down into smaller, more manageable components. Focus on what you need to do now to make some progress, even a little bit. Identify one small step and set a time before the end of the day for completing that step.

For example: Following a low-cholesterol diet can be very challenging. The dietician might make it sound easy, but there are lots of steps involved in a big change like that: learning what foods to buy, changing cooking habits, taking time to avoid convenient (but greasy) food. Making those changes for every meal of every day is too much to do all at once. So you might start with just one meal a week. Choose a day that you have some extra time and energy to try something different. Try to think of it as an experiment. Your goal is to learn what works for you rather than to do everything right the first time.

Staying Physically Active

When medical problems limit your physical capabilities, you may have to give up some of your usual forms of recreation. Even if you are physically limited, however, keep yourself going. Physical activity is safe and beneficial for almost everybody, and it's one of the best natural antidepressants.

For example: Your doctor may have been nagging you for months to start some kind of exercise program. By now, thinking about exercise just makes you feel guilty rather than motivated. When you feel completely stuck, it's time to lower your goals. Planning to jog 4 times a week sounds fantastic, but it's probably not realistic. Try to set a goal so low that you can guarantee success—like walking for 5 minutes. Make the goal a specific one so that you can give yourself credit when you finish. As you accomplish smaller goals, you can gradually work up to setting and achieving goals that are more ambitious. If possible, try to find a friend or family member who'll be your partner.

Making Time for Enjoyment

Medical problems can prevent you from doing things you used to enjoy, like hobbies, socializing and recreation. Missing out on these pleasures can definitely affect your mood. Finding other rewarding things to do as substitutes can make a big difference. You may need to be a little creative about this.

Think about the activities you've found most rewarding in the past. If you can't do those things now, try to think of others that might bring you the same kind of satisfaction. The key to getting started on a new activity is to be specific. Choose what you want to do and make a plan for when you'll start. If possible, include a friend or family member in your plan. Start with a few small things—like listening to music you used to enjoy, or brief get-togethers with friends.

Tom's story:

I developed my depression after learning that I had a degenerative eye disease. The doctor said that limiting my reading would help me retain my eyesight. But that was a real blow. I simply loved to read. A friend reminded me that many books were now on audiotape and others were available in extra large print. After talking to my librarian, I was able to send away for several audiotapes and found I enjoyed this medium almost as much as reading.

Chapter 17 includes more ideas about finding time for enjoyable activities.

Understanding Your Medications

You can never be too well informed about the medicines you're taking, and keeping track of several different ones can be overwhelming.

Learning more about the medicines you're taking and coming up with a sensible schedule for taking them can increase your sense of control over your life. It's especially important to know which ones you should take on a regular schedule and which you can take according to how you feel. Many people find that using a plastic case with small compartments for each day of the week helps them keep track. Such cases are available at most pharmacies.

Finding Support

Becoming an expert manager of your own health and health care takes time. You'll need both lots of knowledge and lots of confidence. You might as well take advantage of what other people have learned along the way. There are probably support groups in your area for people with chronic illnesses like diabetes, arthritis, or heart disease. Ask your doctor or try the telephone book or internet.

You also may need to ask for more help from family or friends. That's not easy for anyone, and it's especially hard if you're feeling depressed and down on yourself. You may want to start slowly and build up your confidence. Experiment with a few small requests. You'll probably be surprised at how much most people appreciate the opportunity to help out.

DEPRESSION TREATMENT FOR PEOPLE WITH CHRONIC ILLNESSES

Antidepressant Medication

Antidepressant medications help to restore the natural balance of essential neurotransmitters (or chemical messengers) such as serotonin or norepinephrine. Antidepressants help with a wide range of physical and mental symptoms including sad or depressed mood, fatigue, loss of interest in activities, sleep problems, and difficulty concentrating. It's important to remember that antidepressants work slowly (over 2 to 3 weeks) and that they work only if you take them every day.

Having a chronic illness doesn't necessarily make it dangerous or more difficult to use antidepressant medications. While antidepressants may have side effects (like upset stomach or dry mouth), these effects are not dangerous or permanent. Of course, your doctor should be aware of other medications you are taking. And your health history may affect what medication your doctor recommends.

One type of medication may be better for people with pain problems while another might be better for people with heart disease.

If you're already taking several medications, adding another to the list may not sound attractive. You and your doctor will have to weigh the pros and cons of starting a new treatment. There may be drawbacks, but the benefits of antidepressant medications can be surprising—especially if you were convinced that fatigue and hopelessness were problems you were stuck with forever.

Chapter 5 includes more information about antidepressants in general, and the Appendix gives details about specific medications.

Counseling or Psychotherapy

If a chronic illness like diabetes or arthritis is your biggest challenge, you may wonder how counseling or psychotherapy can help you. No amount of talking will make arthritis or heart disease go away. But counseling isn't about changing reality, it's about helping you to manage the reality you're stuck with.

Counseling for depression usually focuses on

- increasing your involvement in pleasant or rewarding activities
- learning to identify and "tone down" negative or self-critical thoughts

- effective strategies for solving problems that make you depressed or discouraged

Of course, those are things that are good for you whether you suffer from depression or not. And skills you learn in counseling can certainly help you in managing a chronic illness like diabetes or arthritis.

Chapter 6 includes more specific information about psychotherapy for depression.

Working with Your Health Care Providers

Getting treatment for depression may involve new treatments (like antidepressant medications) from your current health care providers or relationships with new providers, like a counselor or psychiatrist. As usual, you want to make sure that your health care providers communicate with each other and that each one is aware of decisions that another has made. If your providers are part of the same clinic or health care system, that communication may be automatic. If not, keeping the communication open may require some extra effort on your part. Be sure to bring a list of all the medications you take to any doctor visit. If you have questions, don't hesitate to ask. If you are concerned that some treatments might conflict with each other, ask your doctors to talk to each other.

CHAPTER 12

Depression and Women's Health

I'm on my feet all day at my job at the hospital, then I run errands on my way home. When I get there I deal with dinner and laundry and the kids' homework, baths and bedtimes, and then I check in with my elderly dad who lives nearby. I'm so ragged at the end of the day that I collapse into bed. I get tired and overwhelmed so easily these days. I wonder if it is menopause, on top of everything?

For many of us, our lives today seem busier than ever. The stresses and strains of work and family life demand much of our time and energy, and it often is difficult to make time for relaxation and enjoyment. For many women in particular, the tension between the demands of family and/or work roles and good self-care may contribute to depression, anxiety, or a host of stress-related illnesses.

Studies have consistently shown that women are at higher risk for major depression over their lifetimes compared to men. The vulnerability for this extra risk seems to be related to social and biological factors. For some women, managing their conflicting roles as mother, wife, wage earner, housekeeper, and emotional anchor for the family can be stressful. Still other women report that they are sensitive to changes in their hormone levels, finding that they are more susceptible to mood changes at certain times than at others. Women who understand the interaction of these biological and social forces are in a better position to cope with depression when it occurs.

SOCIAL SUPPORT AND DEPRESSION

Relationships are important to women, and the quality of these relationships often determines how they feel about themselves and those they care about. Women who are not in supportive environments, who receive disrespectful treatment from others, or who are socially isolated may not feel that their emotional needs are being met.

Take an inventory of the important relationships in your life. Are there people you should be spending more time with? Others with whom less time might be better? Are there relationships that are important to you but sometimes leave you feeling disappointed? Do the people who are important to you respect you and care for you? Sometimes discussing these relationships with a counselor or a leader in your faith community may help resolve any imbalance you feel.

DEPRESSION AND THE MENSTRUAL CYCLE

Many women report physical and emotional changes that occur prior to their menses. These can range from weight gain and minor irritability to severe negative moods that can even involve thoughts of hopelessness and helplessness. These symptoms, which often appear after ovulation (i.e., generally after the first 15 days of a woman's menstrual cycle) but before the onset of menstruation, are known as PMS, or *premenstrual syndrome*. For some women, these symptoms are very challenging and disabling.

Your doctor may have suggestions for how to cope with your mood swings. Both counseling and antidepressants have been shown to be effective in treating mood swings. Diet, exercise, and changes in your daily routine may also help you cope with these times of increased sensitivity to stress.

ORAL CONTRACEPTIVES

Many women who use oral contraceptives report that their mood is better after starting on these medications, whereas others claim that they are more prone to depression while on these medications.

If your mood becomes more depressed after starting the pill, you may find it helpful to discuss this with your doctor and explore alternative contraceptive methods (either another pill or a nonpill form) that are less likely to cause this problem. Your doctor may also advise you to take extra vitamins (particularly vitamin B6) while you are on the pill since some women have benefited from doing so.

DEPRESSION AFTER CHILDBIRTH

Almost two-thirds of women report feeling blue and depressed for a period of a few days following delivery. These mood changes are probably due to the hormonal changes occurring after delivery. This period of "baby blues" is quite common and is often resolved with the supportive care of family and loved ones. Some women, however, have a more severe and lasting form of postpartum depression that may require medical help. Fortunately, both antidepressant medications and psychotherapy have been shown to be effective treatments for postpartum depression.

Many options are available for women who experience postpartum depression. Be sure to tell your doctor or midwife about your mood problems. A national organization known as Depression After Delivery has local resources that you may find helpful if your depression persists (for more information, see the Resource Guide at the back of this book).

MENOPAUSE

Over the last century, the human life span has steadily increased to the point where most women spend more than a third of their life after menopause. The gradual waning of the menstrual cycle is often associated with hot flashes, sleep problems, mood swings, and irritability. Interestingly, many of these common changes around menopause are similar to symptoms of depression.

Hormone replacement therapy is a common issue many women discuss with their physicians. Scientific findings on benefits and risks of hormone replacement therapy change rapidly. Many women find it difficult to sort through these constantly changing reports on osteoporosis, heart disease, breast cancer, and menopause. There is a workbook available that provides information on the benefits and risks of taking hormone replacement therapy, helps individuals assess their risks, and discusses alternative approaches to relieving menopausal symptoms. It was developed by the Center for Disease Control and the Group Health Cooperative Center for Health Studies and is titled *To Be or Not to Be— On Hormone Replacement Therapy: A Workbook to Help You Explore Your Options* (for more information, see the Resource Guide at the back of this book). You may want to consult your health care provider for the most current recommendations.

Another factor to consider is that many women who have had problems with depression either before or during menopause find that hormone replacement diminishes their mood problems and enhances their sleep, memory, and clarity of thought. It may also promote better sexual enjoyment. However, it's important to remember that if you continue to have depression even after hormone replacement treatment has relieved your menopausal symptoms, you may want to seek treatment for depression.

GETTING GOOD ADVICE

If you feel that any of these biological or social factors are playing a role in your depression, a good place to begin exploring ways to improve your mood, memory, and/or energy level is by discussing your concerns with your doctor. There are many options you can take to alleviate your depression or decrease your sensitivity to the risk factors for depression, including finding support, seeing a counselor, and taking medications. Your doctor's office can offer you referrals and educational material to help you get started. Please consider taking that first step if you feel down or moody and would like to feel better.

CHAPTER 13

Food, Alcohol, and Drugs

I'm the type who will eat to solve problems. It's not possible to think of nutrition when I'm depressed. But I know food doesn't fix emotional problems.

EATING AND APPETITE

Clinical depression changes more than just your mood. It also can affect appetite. Serotonin, one of the chemical messengers involved in depression, helps regulate the sense of fullness after eating. When depression alters the level of serotonin, it can also disrupt appetite.

Some depressed people lose their appetites. No food tastes good. Eating seems like more trouble than it's worth. These people may lose significant amounts of weight. This can be unhealthy or dangerous, particularly in older people.

Other depressed people gain weight. No matter how much they eat, they never feel full. Eating may be one of their few pleasures, so depressed people may eat much more than their bodies need, often in the form of junk food or other empty calories. Overeating can have a negative effect on chronic illnesses such as diabetes and heart disease.

Antidepressants and Appetite

Antidepressants can also affect appetite. In fact, weight gain is one reason some people stop taking antidepressants too soon. This side effect can be so disturbing that some people will quit using an antidepressant even when it is providing significant relief from depression. About 20% of people who take tricyclic antidepressants gain weight. Fortunately, antidepressant medications that increase serotonin (SRIs) are less likely to cause weight gain.

Tricyclic antidepressants may stimulate a chemical reaction that produces a craving for sweets. If you are taking one of these medicines, you may get the urge for cookies, cake, and candy. If you find this to be a problem, or if you gain weight while taking an antidepressant, you should discuss your concerns with your doctor.

Do Certain Foods Reduce Depression?

There is no hard scientific evidence pointing to specific foods that can help lift your mood when you are depressed.

Even if you're not hungry, eat regular meals. Avoid caffeinated foods and drinks such as chocolate, coffee, and cola because you're likely to feel a letdown after the stimulating effect of the caffeine wears off.

VITAMINS AND NUTRIENTS

Many depressed people wonder if vitamins might give them back their lost energy. In general, the answer is no. Depression is rarely due to a nutritional deficiency. However, the vitamins most often deficient in depressed people are folate (sometimes called folacin or folic acid) and, to a lesser degree, B12. Folate is found in leafy green vegetables. B12 is found in meat. If you do not eat these foods, you may want to talk to your doctor about whether you should be taking a supplement.

Try to follow these simple guidelines if you experience a change in appetite:

- If you're not hungry, at least choose what your body needs most. This includes water (some experts recommend eight glasses a day) and wholesome foods like fruits, vegetables, and whole grains

- If you're eating too much, at least try to avoid what your body doesn't need. This includes foods with empty calories such as chips and sweets.

ALCOHOL

Depressed people are typically anxious, restless, and short on sleep. To relieve those problems, people sometimes turn to alcohol. Many people rely on beer, wine, or hard liquor to relax at the end of the day or on the weekend. It seems to raise their spirits, at least while they are drinking it. But the benefits of drinking are brief, and the problems it creates can last a long time.

When you drink, your mood tends to improve only as long as your blood level of alcohol is rising. This is the early phase. But as the amount of alcohol in your blood goes down, so does your mood. In fact, during this phase your mood can go down further than it was before you took a drink, leaving you even more depressed. This is one reason why people who drink when they are depressed are more likely to commit suicide than those who do not drink.

Tolerance and Physical Dependence

If you drink alcohol regularly, you will develop tolerance to its effects. That means you must drink more and more in order to feel the same intoxication you felt when you first began to drink.

Regular drinking can also make you physically dependent on alcohol. Your body becomes so adjusted to drinking alcohol that it will go into withdrawal if you stop. Withdrawal from chronic drinking can induce seizures, hallucinations, and DTs (delirium tremens), which can be fatal.

Alcohol and Antidepressants Don't Mix

Alcohol does not mix with antidepressants. If you drink while taking your medicine, you will feel roughly twice as drunk per drink as you would normally.

In addition, regular use of alcohol, in small amounts, keeps antidepressants from working. It's best not to drink any alcohol while you are just beginning to take antidepressants. After a week or two, it may be all right to have an occasional glass of beer or wine with dinner, but you should avoid heavier use of alcohol.

If you aren't sure if you should have an occasional drink, check with your doctor or pharmacist. Most containers of prescription antidepressants come with a label warning against drinking while taking the medication.

Risks Outweigh the Benefits

People who are depressed should avoid drinking alcohol for the following reasons:

- Trying to treat your depression symptoms with alcohol can cause you to postpone getting the kind of treatment that will really help you feel better.
- Drinking can increase the risk of suicide, both while you are drinking and afterward, when your mood worsens.
- Excessive use of alcohol also decreases your ability to understand your situation clearly. It does nothing to

solve the problems in your life. It does not help you learn how to deal with disappointment and frustration.

- Although alcohol may initially help you fall asleep, you're likely to wake up again in 2–4 hours, when the level of alcohol in your blood drops, and have difficulty getting back to sleep.
- Alcohol can worsen chronic medical illnesses, such as diabetes, by raising blood glucose levels.

ILLEGAL DRUGS

Depression can cause some people who don't normally use illegal drugs to consider trying them. Relief may seem worth the risk. Unfortunately, using these drugs involves the same psychological risks as drinking alcohol.

Marijuana

Some people claim marijuana and hashish can decrease anxiety or insomnia. In fact, some people may experience short-term benefits. In other people, however, marijuana can cause feelings of paranoia. A person in a paranoid state becomes extremely suspicious of other people, and the fear associated with feelings of paranoia can be intense.

Marijuana can also produce panic attacks. During panic attacks, intense fears of dying or going crazy combine with physical symptoms such as shortness of breath, pounding heart, nausea, sweating, shaking, or numbness. These severe reactions usually wear off as the marijuana wears off, but not always.

People who use marijuana also sleep less deeply. The morning after using marijuana, people tend to feel less refreshed than they do normally. In addition, marijuana can often damage your memory and rob you of motivation.

Stimulants

Stimulants are powerful drugs such as cocaine or amphetamines that elevate the mood even of severely depressed people. However, these mood-lifting effects are short-lived. The crash after a binge on cocaine or crack cocaine can be devastating. Cocaine users try to avoid this awful letdown by continuing to use the drug for as long as possible. But eventually they have to come down. When they do, they are at increased risk for suicide. Stimulants should not be mixed with antidepressants because they deplete the same brain chemicals that antidepressants are working to restore.

Part II

EVERYDAY INSIGHTS

What to Expect in This Section

Insights on

- Social and physical activity
- Sleep and its impact on mood
- Upward and downward "spirals"
- Setting up a support system; reaching out for help

FACT
Without medication, the chances of a bout of depression returning are 50% after one episode, 70% after two episodes, and 90% after three episodes.
—American Family Physician

PRACTICAL TIPS FOR COPING WITH DEPRESSION
Try to exercise more* / Plan activities that allow for social interaction / Consider getting a pet / Reach out to old and new friends, family, neighbors / Get away for a weekend / Get involved in your community

* Always consult your physician before starting an exercise program because certain kinds of physical activity can be harmful for those with specific medical conditions.

CHAPTER 14

Relaxing

At the end of the workday, I'm so tense my shoulders are up to my ears! I'm like a rubber band—ready to snap.

TENSION AND DEPRESSION

Tension is what happens to your body when you are under stress. Tension gets in the way of doing the things that help you overcome depression. Trying out a new activity, or speaking assertively to someone, can make you tense. And sometimes the hassles of everyday life make it difficult to avoid feeling tense. Unfortunately, feeling tense can reduce the levels of key chemicals in the brain, thereby triggering or sustaining depression.

Many of us get caught up in a cycle of working too hard and too long without breaks for fun and relaxation. Sometimes doing anything other than intense work makes us worry and feel guilty. But taking time for relaxation and leisure can actually lead to a more productive and enjoyable work life. Achieving a balance between the things you must do and the things that give you peace of mind and body will pay off in both the short- and the long-term.

Various relaxation techniques can help you relieve the tension that builds up from the day-to-day stresses of a busy life. It may sound odd, but relaxation takes effort, not just plopping down in front of the TV.

SIMPLE STEPS TO RELIEVING TENSION

Some tension-reducing activities are simple and don't require new skills. Easy activities such as the following may help ease your tension:

- Listening to music
- Taking a warm bath or shower
- Getting a massage
- Following a yoga or exercise routine
- Rocking in a rocking chair
- Drinking a cup of herbal tea
- Going for a walk

The key to learning how to relax is to practice relaxation techniques regularly. Set specific times and places for relaxing. Arrange to be free from distractions that compete for your attention. Take the phone off the hook. Close your bedroom door if the kids are watching television. Some tension-reducing activities may take a bit of practice before they feel comfortable and easy. You will soon enjoy your daily relaxation time so much that it will become a habit.

DEEP MUSCLE RELAXATION

Deep muscle relaxation can teach you how to recognize tension in different muscle groups and how to systematically release that tension.

Deep muscle relaxation involves first tensing and then relaxing different muscle groups in your body. Once you can do this, muscle tension will become a cue or reminder for you to relax. When you have learned deep muscle relaxation, you'll be able to relax yourself at the first signs of tension.

When you are first learning this technique, you may want to use one of many widely available audiotapes that can guide you through the deep muscle relaxation procedure. After a few run-throughs you won't need the tape, although you may still want to use it to cue your body to relax or as part of a soothing bedtime ritual.

Here's how to do deep muscle relaxation:

In a quiet and moderately lit room, sit in a comfortable chair that supports your entire body. Loosen your clothes and take off your shoes. Position yourself comfortably in the chair and take several deep breaths. Begin by focusing on the muscles in your shoulders. Crunch your shoulders up toward your ears, making them tense and tight for 5 seconds. Focus on the feeling of tension. After 5 seconds release your shoulders totally, noticing the difference in how your shoulders feel in both positions. Pay attention to how your shoulders feel when they're fully relaxed. Repeat, first tensing your shoulder muscles for a few seconds, then relaxing them again fully. Continue tensing and relaxing different muscle groups one at time. Tense and relax your face, neck, shoulders, arms, hands, abdomen, back, buttocks, thighs, calves, and feet. In each session, go through each muscle group twice before moving on to tense and relax the next body part.

BREATHING: THE GREAT ARMCHAIR ESCAPE

The armchair escape will help you focus on your breathing and shift your breathing from shallow to deep. This breathing technique can help you relax when you don't have time to practice the full routine of deep muscle relaxation. You can do it any time, any place.

1. Let your shoulders drop.
2. Breathe in as slowly and deeply as you can through your nose.
3. Hold your breath while you count to four.

4. Breathe out slowly until you've emptied all the air from your lungs.

5. Repeat five times.

MEDITATION AND RELAXING IMAGERY

Meditation and imagery can both help ease your tension and quiet your mind. Meditation involves focusing all your thoughts on a particular word, sound, or image. Imagery is picturing yourself in a very relaxed setting. You may want to try each one, and see which you like better.

Meditation

Close your eyes and focus your mind on a single soothing word (such as "relax"), a single sound (such as that of a waterfall), or a single image (such as a full moon). Keep your mind focused on that word, sound, or image. When you find your thoughts drifting to something else, gently return your thoughts to the original word, sound, or image. Practice this for a few minutes at first, working up to 15 minutes.

Imagery

Close your eyes and imagine yourself in a relaxing place—lying on a sunny beach or in a meadow, strolling by a babbling brook or hanging in a hammock in a cozy room. Imagine this scene using all your senses. What do you see?

What do you hear? What do you smell? What do you feel on your skin? Stay with the scene for 10 or 15 minutes or until you feel ready to return to your real surroundings.

Most community centers, such as YMCAs and YWCAs, offer inexpensive classes on relaxation, meditation or yoga. You can learn these skills on your own from books or videotapes, but many people find that classes provide the structure and social reinforcement necessary to learn a new skill.

STRETCHING

Stretching can help ease physical tension, increase flexibility, and prevent and lessen backaches and other pain.

- Take 2-*minute breaks* during the day, to stretch your neck, back, shoulders, and legs. You can also stretch first thing in the morning to help prepare for your day, or in front of the television to unwind at the end of the day.
- *Videotapes or books*, for rent or purchase, can teach effective ways to safely stretch the parts of your body that are particularly tight and tense. When you begin, stretch slowly and only as far as is comfortable without bouncing. While breathing deeply, hold each stretch for several seconds.

CHAPTER 15

Exercising

I've always been very active and love to run, but then I injured my back. I tried other things, but nothing made me feel as good as running. Slowly, I'm starting to jog again.

WHY EXERCISE?

People who exercise regularly feel calmer and happier, concentrate better, sleep more soundly, have higher self-esteem, and are less irritable and anxious.

Researchers have found that exercise improves mood in several different ways. Exercise increases the blood levels of *endorphins*, the body's own painkillers, which may improve mood. Exercise also affects the same mood-altering chemical messengers that antidepressants target. Because the chemical consequences of exercise and antidepressants are similar, exercising while taking an antidepressant may boost the medicine's effectiveness.

If you have never exercised regularly, this may seem like a strange time to start. Your energy may be low. You may think it's unlikely that exercise could help you feel better. But try to set aside your doubts. No matter how tired you are, your fatigue will usually lift after some aerobic or stretching exercises. Give exercise a chance for several weeks.

For exercise to help, you should find an activity that you will enjoy and stick with over the long run. And you have a lot of options. Exercise can be solitary or social, self-directed or competitive, slow-paced or vigorous, depending on your preference. If you're not already exercising regularly, begin this week and see how it goes.

Some people believe that the physical and mental-health benefits of exercise can be achieved only if you work up a good sweat. How many times have you heard someone say, "No pain, no gain?" But nonstrenuous exercise like going for a walk or working in the garden can help reduce stress and improve your mood.

MAKING AN EXERCISE PLAN

Exercise works best if you do it regularly. People who exercise regularly often have an exercise plan. A plan means choosing a time and place for exercise, selecting a specific exercise activity, and sometimes persuading a friend to join you.

The first step in putting together an exercise plan is to determine your present level of fitness. If you are older than 50 or have any chronic medical problems, consult with your doctor before beginning a strenuous exercise program. Almost anyone can begin walking right away, however.

You can usually determine your fitness level by trying something simple like walking or jogging. For several days in a row, walk or jog until you begin to feel tired. Whatever distance and speed you can do repeatedly without feeling tired is your baseline level. This is where you should start. Don't worry if you can't do much at first. The benefits of exercise are actually the greatest for people who start from a very low level.

The second step is to design an exercise schedule. It's not necessary to exercise every day. Three times a week is plenty. Pick activities you like. For example:

- Take a walk, by yourself or with a friend.
- Ride a stationary bicycle while watching TV.
- Walk up and down stairs while listening to music.
- Take an aerobics class in your neighborhood.
- Join a local league to play a competitive sport such as soccer, volleyball, or tennis.

It's okay if you don't stick with your schedule completely. You may intend to walk a half-hour every day, but then miss 3 days in a row. Don't think that all is lost. Just get back to your exercise routine as soon as you can. If you've missed more than a week, you may need to start at a lower level and work your way up to where you were when you stopped.

WHAT TO EXPECT FROM EXERCISE

- Your body and your mind both need exercise. Start slowly, though. Regular moderate exercise is more important than big changes in activity level. Avoid a boom-and-bust cycle in which you exercise very hard then rest for many days because you're so tired and sore. Patience will pay off.
- You may notice you're feeling calmer and more energetic after only a week of regular exercise, or it may take a few months for your mood to change. It requires some dedication to get over this hump.
- Many people who start a regular exercise program never stop. Once you get used to exercising, it could become one of the highlights of your day.

CHAPTER 16

Getting a Good Night's Sleep

When I was depressed, I'd lie in bed awake and think.
Nothing important, but I'd just lie there like my body was
sleeping but my eyes were open.

YOUR NATURAL SLEEP CYCLE

Your body has its own biological clock that regulates your
activity and alertness. When this clock is on schedule, your
body slows down naturally for sleep at night and speeds
up again in the morning. But depression disrupts this natural clock. It interrupts your sleep and makes you feel restless because your body is getting mixed messages about
whether it's daytime or nighttime.

Your sleep rhythm can also be upset by circumstances
other than your depression, such as medical problems,

pain, alcohol or drugs, late-night coffee drinking, or changes in your sleep schedule. Any of these can interact with depression and make your symptoms worse.

DOs AND DON'Ts FOR RESTFUL SLEEP

Don't Use Caffeine

When your sleep cycle is already upset, even small amounts of caffeine can interfere with restful sleep. The best amount of caffeine is none. If you feel you can't give it up completely, limit yourself to one cup of coffee in the morning. Be sure to avoid caffeine in the late afternoon or evening. And remember that some soft drinks contain caffeine, as does chocolate. You may be tempted to pick yourself up with caffeine after a poor night's sleep, but it's best to avoid those caffeine jolts to your system.

Don't Drink Alcohol

Alcohol's effects on sleep can be deceiving. Alcohol has a relaxing effect for the first few hours, but once this sedation wears off, you'll feel more anxious and jittery. If you drink in the evening, you may find yourself waking in the middle of the night. Regular drinking can make sleep problems worse. If you're having trouble sleeping, don't try to use alcohol to bring on sleep.

Do Exercise

Regular exercise can help restore your normal sleep pattern. Even walking for only 20 to 30 minutes several times a week will help. Try not to exercise close to bedtime: evening exercise can leave you feeling too charged up to fall asleep easily.

Do Establish a Bedtime Routine

Setting up a regular procedure for retiring is one way of telling your biological clock, "It's time for bed now." Slow down as bedtime approaches. Stick to quiet, relaxing activities for at least an hour beforehand.

RESETTING YOUR BIOLOGICAL CLOCK

When your natural sleep cycle is disturbed, it may have trouble resetting itself. The solution is to stick with a healthy sleeping schedule. Make yourself stay on schedule for a week or two, and your own natural rhythm will usually reestablish itself. Try following these steps:

Set a Regular Waking Time and Stick with It

The key to restoring a healthy schedule is setting a regular time to get up each morning. Your waking time is the signal that allows your biological clock to reset itself. Choose a time that works for you, and get up at that time no matter what. Even if you slept poorly the night before, adhere to your schedule. Sleeping late to make up for a bad night's sleep upsets your own internal rhythm.

At first, you will probably need to set a time for going to bed as well. To do so, start with your wake-up time and move back 7 or 8 hours (or whatever your normal sleep time is). After a while, your body will tell you when you need to go to sleep. If you stick by your waking time, bedtime should take care of itself.

Try Not to Vary from Day to Day

Shifting your schedule back and forth sends mixed messages to your biological clock. Don't sleep late on weekends or holidays. When you're having trouble sleeping, it's best not to vary your schedule more than an hour. Once your sleep cycle is reestablished, you may be able to give yourself a little more leeway.

Avoid Daytime Naps

Taking a nap during the day tells your biological clock, "It's nighttime now." Even when you're having trouble sleeping at night, don't take daytime naps. Concentrate your sleep where it ought to be: at night.

You May Sleep Better by Sleeping Less

People tend to need less sleep as they get older. Of course, the amount of sleep needed in a 24-hour period varies from person to person. Some people may be programmed to sleep 4 or 5 hours a night while others do better with 8 or more.

Whatever amount of sleep is best for you, you'll probably feel more rested if you get it all at once. If you lie in bed for 10 hours but only sleep 6, you're likely to get up exhausted. You'll feel better if you get those same 6 hours of sleep during a 7-hour period.

If your sleep is interrupted and restless, try cutting down on the amount of time in bed. You'll probably spend just as many hours sleeping, but fewer hours tossing and turning.

"LEARNED" INSOMNIA (AND HOW TO UNLEARN IT)

Lying awake at night can be self-reinforcing: the longer you fret about going back to sleep, the more awake you feel. Often the most disturbing part of insomnia is the time you spend worrying about it. After several nights of lying awake, your mind comes to associate lying in bed with staying awake and worrying, exactly the opposite of what you want! Stop trying so hard. Sleep can't be forced.

If You Lie in Bed Unable to Sleep for More Than 20 Minutes:

• Get up and go to another room.
• Do something quiet and relaxing.

- When you feel sleepy, go back to bed.

You may worry that you'll miss too much sleep this way. Actually, you'll probably feel more rested.

About Sleeping Pills

Sleeping pills can help you sleep, but only for a short while. Sleeping medication can reduce the time it takes to fall asleep and time spent awake during the night. After 2 or 3 weeks of regular use, however, your body adjusts to the drug's effects. This causes two problems. First, the medication doesn't work as well (and you may be tempted to take more). Second, when you try to stop, you may go through a period of even worse insomnia or anxiety—a withdrawal reaction known as *rebound insomnia*. Used regularly, sleeping pills can also depress your mood, reduce your energy, and disrupt your memory and concentration. Because these effects build up slowly over time, you might not realize what the medication is doing.

Your doctor may prescribe sleeping pills, to be used for a brief period. If you still feel you need sleeping pills after 2 weeks, discuss the situation with your doctor.

ANTIDEPRESSANTS AND SLEEP

Antidepressants can improve your sleep in two ways. First, some antidepressants have a sedative effect. These should improve your sleeping in just a few days (sometimes after just the first dose). If you are taking one of these antidepressants, try taking it an hour before bedtime. Second, antidepressants restore normal sleep cycles by increasing the levels of chemical messengers in the brain. This leads to more restful sleep. It may take a few weeks before you notice this effect, but most people report significant improvement in their sleep.

Occasionally an antidepressant interferes with sleeping because in some people it acts as a stimulant. If you notice this reaction, try taking your antidepressant in the morning. If the new schedule doesn't help, or if the effect is severe, check with your doctor about reducing the dose or changing to a different antidepressant.

CHAPTER 17

Making Time for Enjoyment

I've lightened the load, and that enables me to enjoy life more. I used to think that was selfish, but now I realize it's a lot healthier. Before, I felt I couldn't do things. Now I try even if I'm not sure I'll be able to. You can at least try.

AVOIDING THE DOWNWARD SPIRAL

People who feel depressed usually stop doing the things that once brought them pleasure. This cycle of worsening depression is sometimes called a *negative downward spiral* (Figure 17-1).

Making time for pleasure and reward in your life can help you reverse a downward spiral into a *positive upward spiral*. You will also feel better when you are successful at something.

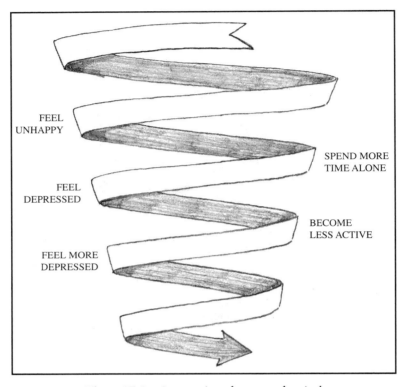

FEEL
UNHAPPY

SPEND MORE
TIME ALONE

FEEL
DEPRESSED

BECOME
LESS ACTIVE

FEEL MORE
DEPRESSED

Figure 17-1—A negative downward spiral

"Easier said than done," you might think, feeling like you have barely enough energy to push the buttons on the TV remote. But it really is true that participating in positive activities can break a negative cycle and turn a negative spiral into a positive upward spiral (Figure 17-2).

Often the hardest part is getting started. Antidepressant medications may boost your energy level and make it easier to start being more active. With or without antide-

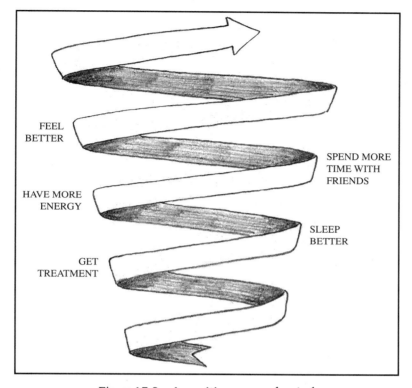

FEEL
BETTER

SPEND MORE
TIME WITH
FRIENDS

HAVE MORE
ENERGY

SLEEP
BETTER

GET
TREATMENT

Figure 17-2—A positive upward spiral

pressants, though, it's true that what you do affects the way you feel.

FEELINGS, THOUGHTS, AND ACTIONS

You can think of your mental state as a three-part system that is made up of feelings, thoughts, and actions. All three parts interact to affect each other (Figure 17-3). For

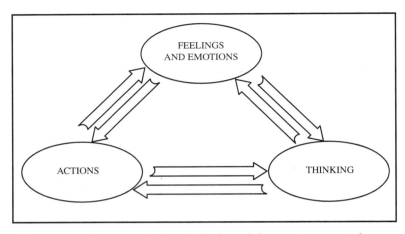

Figure 17-3—How you feel and think and the actions you take are all related to one another.

example, how you feel affects how you think and behave, which then affects how you feel and think—and so on.

When they are depressed, many people think they should be trying to change their emotions, since their emotions seem to be where they are having problems. But emotions are not readily controlled. It's actually much easier to change your actions and thoughts. Believe it or not, changing what you do and what you think will, in turn, change how you feel.

Some Effective Activities

The two types of activities that are particularly effective in changing your emotions to reduce depression are *pleasant social activities* and *successful activities*.

- *Pleasant social activities* are the enjoyable times that you spend with other people, especially friends and family.
- *Successful activities* are experiences that give you a sense of accomplishment and pride, whether it's completing a tough project at work or adding an extra 4 blocks to your usual walk. When you feel you have done something well, your self-confidence goes up. You're also more likely to do other things, which in turn makes you feel even better.

PLANNING TO HAVE A BETTER TIME

When you are depressed, it often seems easier and less frightening to do nothing. Fear, anxiety, and apathy are all common feelings among people who are depressed. But you don't have to do much. Just plan one small pleasant activity every day.

Begin by scheduling one short, enjoyable event for each day in the upcoming week. Think of some activities you used to enjoy. Perhaps there are also some new activities that you would like to try.

Ideally, they should be

- Activities you truly enjoy
- Activities you can do frequently
- Activities that are relatively inexpensive

- Activities you feel you can control
- Activities that will not upset others

Examples of pleasurable activities might include

- Reading a book or magazine
- Listening to music
- Drinking a cup of tea
- Taking a walk with a friend
- Planning or organizing an event
- Skating, bicycling, or swimming
- Writing a letter to a friend
- Looking through old family photographs
- Browsing in a hardware or antique store
- Watching a videotape
- Being with dogs, cats, or other pets
- Talking to a friend on the phone
- Gardening or doing yard work
- Planning a trip or vacation
- Having lunch with friends
- Taking a drive to the beach or mountains

Remember, this isn't an unnecessary indulgence: it's something you need to do to make yourself feel better. It may help if some of your plans include another person. This may help prevent you from backing out or making excuses when you're feeling ambivalent.

Get into the habit of scheduling your pleasant activities in advance. You can set aside blocks of time in your daily planner or calendar for things you want to do as well as the things you must do. Your goal is to achieve a better balance between the "wants" and the "musts" in your life.

Planning for Better Living

Use the "Planning for Better Living" worksheet that we have provided to help you build rewarding activities into your life every day. You might try out the technique on a small activity before tackling a really challenging one.

MAKING TIME FOR ENJOYMENT

1. What are some pleasurable activities you have enjoyed in the past?

_____

_____

_____

2. What would be enjoyable to do right now?

_____

_____

_____

3. What social activities could you plan to arrange this week?

_____

_____

_____

4. What small thing could you do today that would be an accomplishment for you?

_____

_____

_____

Additional copies of this worksheet are located at the back of the book.

CHAPTER 18

Thinking More Constructively

I've learned to listen to my thoughts, determining how true
they are and discarding the erroneous ones. Telling myself
I'm stupid doesn't help. What does help is reviewing what's
happened, figuring out what went wrong, and putting a
plan in place to prevent it from happening again.

CONSTRUCTIVE THINKING REDUCES DEPRESSION

Everyone has negative thoughts once in a while. But if your negative thoughts occur too frequently, you'll feel down all the time.

The first step in developing more constructive thinking is to identify your frequent negative thoughts (Figure 18-1). Here are some examples of negative thoughts that may sound familiar:

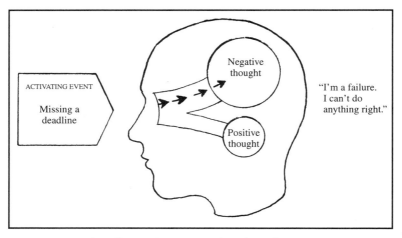

Figure 18-1—Negative thoughts

- Nobody loves me.
- What's the use?
- I'm worthless.
- It's all my fault.
- I can't cope with this pain anymore.
- Why do bad things always happen to me?
- I'll never get over this depression.
- I am not as good as Mary.
- I can't think of anything to do that would be fun.

A negative thought is usually caused by some situation or event. This situation or event is called an *activating event* or a *trigger event*. For example, suppose you miss a bus on the way to work in the morning. A negative thought that

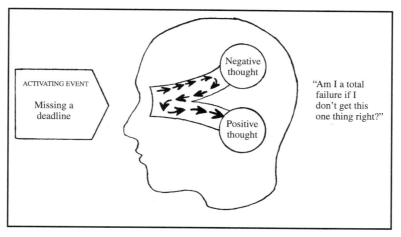

Figure 18-2—Rerouting negative thoughts

might follow this activating event is "I can't do anything right; I can't even get to the bus on time."

One key to overcoming depression is to fight off negative thoughts when they occur (Figure 18-2).

One way to begin thinking more constructively is to substitute a positive counter thought for this negative thought (Figure 18-3). A positive counter thought is a more realistic, and usually optimistic, thought about the same activating event.

Many of the thoughts that make you feel bad are irrational. Negative thoughts are often overreactions in which you exaggerate the circumstances, impose unrealistic expectations on yourself or someone else, or jump to conclusions.

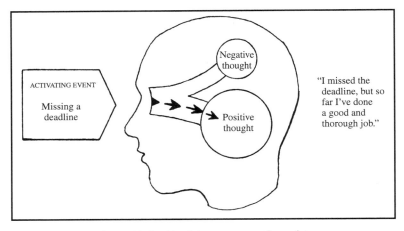

Figure 18-3—Positive counterthoughts

Stephanie's story:

I asked a coworker to lunch. The coworker said she couldn't go because she was too busy. I thought, "She must not like me. I'll probably never have lunch with her again." I felt rejected.

Terry's story:

When my coworker told me she was too busy to go to lunch, I thought, "'Well, we can go to lunch another day. She's still my friend."

ARGUING WITH YOUR IRRATIONAL THOUGHTS

Learn to recognize your self-critical thoughts and learn to confront them. Instead of simply accepting the idea that all your thoughts are true, imagine that you're in a debate with yourself. Train yourself to challenge your thoughts, asking just how true they really are. You may be surprised to find that many of the thoughts that have been getting you down are irrational.

People often make grand, irrational generalizations from a single event. But remember: sleeping through a PTA meeting doesn't mean you're a bad parent. Turning in a sloppy report doesn't mean you're lazy and incompetent. Making one mistake does not mean that you're a failure, or that you will never succeed again, or that no one likes you.

Bob's story:

I was in charge of a complicated project at work, and it was going more slowly than I'd planned. My first thought was, "If I don't get this project done by tomorrow, I'm a total failure. Then I thought, "Is this really true? Am I a total failure in everything if I don't get this one project done by a particular date?"

REPLACING NEGATIVE THOUGHTS WITH POSITIVE ONES

Once you are able to identify some of your negative thoughts and discover how they affect your behavior and feelings, it is only a short step to changing your thinking so that it is more constructive.

Bob's story:
I may not have the project done by tomorrow as I'd hoped, but so far I've done a good and thorough job.

ACCEPTING SOME NEGATIVE THOUGHTS

Don't expect all your negative thoughts to go away. You'll still have some; everyone does. Your goal will be to challenge your negative thoughts and take back some control over your thinking. If your self-critical thoughts come back, you'll be able to feel annoyed instead of overwhelmed. Sometimes the best response to such thoughts is, "There you go again!"

TAMING YOUR EXPECTATIONS

Many depressed people have extremely high, and often unrealistic, expectations of themselves. When they don't live up to their own expectations, they blame themselves for failing.

Ed's story:
I still exercise, but I've cut back on how competitive and demanding of myself I am. I had an unrealistic training schedule and also an unrealistic notion of what I could do at my age and for my ability.

TIPS FOR REDUCING NEGATIVE THOUGHTS

Besides challenging and countering irrational thoughts, here are some other useful techniques for helping you short-circuit your negative thinking:

The Rubber-Band Technique

Wear a rubber band on your wrist. Snap it every time you find yourself thinking negative thoughts. It may take a little practice to become adept at recognizing your negative thoughts.

Thought Stopping

When you catch yourself thinking negatively, tell yourself "STOP!" When you are alone, you can even try yelling "STOP!" very loudly. Around other people, you can think, "STOP!" and visualize a stop sign. Say to yourself, "I'm not going to think about this anymore," and switch to thinking about something else. Like the rubber-band technique, this may require a little practice.

Worrying Time

Each week on your calendar, set aside a time and place for worrying and thinking negatively, just the way you schedule times for pleasurable or relaxing activities. Fifteen to twenty minutes should be fine. During this worrying time, do nothing except focus on your worries and negative thoughts; don't watch television, eat, or do anything else. When you catch yourself thinking negatively at other times during the week, remind yourself that this is not your worrying time. Save up those worries and think about them only during the period you have set aside for worrying. This technique may sound silly, but it really works. People who schedule worrying time actually do worry less the rest of the time.

The Buddy System

Tell a friend about a situation that provoked your negative thoughts. Friends can help you sort out and identify the depressing thoughts that are unrealistic and give you support that will also help you feel better.

CHAPTER 19

The Other People in Your Life

I told my closest colleagues at work about my depression and antidepressant medication. Just sharing made me feel better, and it made me understand what it is like to not be isolated. Several of my coworkers also shared with me that they had also been depressed in the past. I no longer felt different.

STRENGTHEN YOUR SUPPORT SYSTEM

When people are depressed, they often don't want to socialize, even with friends and family they ordinarily have fun with. But when you avoid people, you deprive yourself of a source of pleasure, and it's easy to become even more depressed. This leads to doing even fewer things with others, and the cycle continues until you may feel so depressed that you spend most of your time alone.

Even though it seems hard at first, work to strengthen your social support system. The term *social support system* refers to the people in your life (family, friends, coworkers, neighbors, and acquaintances) with whom you have frequent contact and who are on your side. This contact may be in person, through the mail, on the telephone, even via your computer. The important thing is that you have people with whom you can talk freely, feel comfortable, and seek comfort.

Having a strong support system will help you weather tough situations. The people who are part of your support system can do more than just show you they care. They can also help you challenge your negative thinking about yourself, your world, and the future. People with depression tend to be much more critical of themselves than their friends would be.

Keep in mind that antidepressant medication may increase your energy and decrease your irritability, so taking an antidepressant could help improve the time you spend with other people.

INCREASE YOUR CONTACTS WITH FAMILY AND FRIENDS

When you're depressed, socializing can feel like a major effort. You may even wonder who would want to be with you in your present state of mind. Perhaps your most recent contacts with your family and friends have not been pleasant. It may be hard to imagine how spending even more time with them could be rewarding.

One way to get more pleasure from social situations is to make sure that when you're with other people you're doing something you really enjoy. You're more likely to be in a good mood and friendlier to others.

Some Activities You Might Enjoy with Other People Include

- Playing or watching sports
- Cooking
- Getting involved in religious or spiritual groups in your community
- Joining a volunteer group that helps other people
- Taking dancing lessons
- Joining an outdoors club
- Volunteering for a local political or civic group

STAY AWAY FROM FAULT-FINDERS

Decrease your contact with people who always criticize and who regularly bring you down or cause you stress. People with depression are self-critical enough; they don't need help!

BECOME MORE ASSERTIVE

People who are depressed typically have difficulty express-
ing their likes and dislikes. Developing your ability to
express your thoughts and feelings more openly—becoming more assertive—can improve the quality of your contacts with other people.

Four Steps to Becoming More Assertive

1. Decide what you want in a specific situation.
2. Decide what you want to say. Use a personal statement,
    and make your statement short, simple, and clear.
3. Face the person when speaking, and look directly at
    him or her. Make sure your facial expression and tone
    of voice agree with your message.
4. Pick an appropriate place and time to express your
    message.

Being Assertive

You are assertive when you act in your own best interests,
stand up for yourself, and express yourself honestly without putting other people down. Being assertive doesn't
mean things will turn out exactly as you want, but it does
make it more likely you will reach your goal in a satisfac-
tory way.

Example:: I want an appointment with my doctor this week.

Being Passive

You are passive when you fail to act in your own best interests, don't stand up for yourself, and don't honestly say what you think and feel. Being passive makes you feel helpless and controlled because you are unlikely to reach your goals.

Example: Whatever appointment you can give me is fine with me.

Being Aggressive

You are aggressive when you use hostile words or actions to force other people to give in to you. Although you may get what you want, other people may dislike you and try to retaliate.

Example: Are you deaf? I said I want an appointment tomorrow!

Your goal is to be clear about what you want but to be polite and calm as you explain. As you work to stop being passive and timid, don't go too far in the opposite direction and become an aggressive bully.

CHAPTER 20

Intimacy and Sex When You Are Depressed

*I've always enjoyed my sex life, but recently it hasn't been
very satisfying for me or my partner. I just haven't felt like
making love. I feel so tired all the time that sex is the last
thing on my mind. Even when I get aroused enough to
want to have an intimate moment with my partner, I find it
very difficult to achieve orgasm. I feel like it's created a lot of
tension between us, and, although I know my partner still
loves me, our time together just doesn't seem to be the same.*

Depression can create special problems in intimate
sexual relationships. Because depression tends to diminish one's appreciation of pleasurable activities in life, it frequently causes frustration and disappointment in sexual
encounters, leading to decreasing sexual contact and loss
of intimacy. At a time when the depressed person needs

increased support and caring, he or she may have difficulty feeling close to the most important person in his/her world.

MAINTAINING INTIMACY AND SEXUAL CONTACT WITH YOUR PARTNER

When depression is at its worst, sex can be a very low priority. Depressed individuals sometimes feel as though they're barely surviving life, and may have difficulty becoming sexually aroused or maintaining concentration on sensations and experiences that they would usually find stimulating. They may also feel fatigue or a lack of pleasure in general, and may not look forward to sexual encounters even with a loving and gentle partner. Many depressed people have feelings of worthlessness or lowered self-esteem, or beliefs that their bodies are no longer attractive to their partners. Some will "force" themselves to have sex and then become frustrated over inabilities to physically accommodate their partners comfortably. Orgasms may be difficult even with careful prolonged stimulation.

The effects of depression on sex are not limited to the depressed individual. Often the partner will have complex feelings about the relationship. These can range from guilt about asking the depressed partner for intimate contact, selfishness for encouraging a fatigued partner to have sex, or frustration and sadness in watching the depressed individual withdraw from a previously fulfilling aspect of the relationship.

BROADENING YOUR SEXUAL PLEASURE

For humans, sex can be much more than the act of intercourse. People can find enormous pleasure and enjoyment from many other intimate activities. Couples who are highly satisfied with their sex lives often view "sex" as a range of behaviors including kissing, caressing, sexual and intimate talk, exploring each others' bodies, experiencing the taste and smell of their partners, and sharing sexual fantasies as well as intercourse and orgasms.

Depressed individuals often underestimate the amount of sexual interest that can be evoked by skilled and caring partners. Setting limited goals (e.g., sitting together and holding one another with no expectation that sexual intercourse will result) can often set the stage for increasingly intimate experiences where partners do not feel rushed. Time spent together walking, talking, or doing projects frequently deepens the desire for intimacy, which can often be very fulfilling for both partners. Partners can learn to perform sensuous massage and other relaxing experiences that promote closeness. For many people, these intimacy experiences are more important than sexual orgasm. It is important for couples to talk with each other about their expectations. You may find that your partner is less interested in orgasm itself than the process leading up to it.

MEDICATIONS AND SEX

While loss of interest in sexual activity and difficulty in achieving orgasm can be part of depression, they can also be the result of medications used to treat depression. As many as 20% of people taking antidepressants report that their ability to enjoy sex or to achieve orgasm is diminished. Usually this is a temporary or slight decrease, but in some cases it can result in a dramatic decline in interest or ability in a person who was previously sexually well-adjusted.

You need not feel discouraged, however, about taking medications for your depression. There are many ways to deal with this medication side effect, and you can talk with your doctor about your options. Some antidepressants have no negative effects on sexual functioning, and your doctor may suggest that you switch to one of these. The most important consideration is to get your depression under control. For the vast majority of people, the interest in sex will return naturally as they recover.

Above all, remember that although depression may temporarily diminish the quantity and/or quality of the sex that you or your partner enjoy, adherence to treatment and exploration of alternative forms of intimacy will gradually restore the satisfying physical and emotional contact you previously enjoyed in your relationship.

CHAPTER 21

Managing at Work When You Are Depressed

My worst fear was that I would lose my job. I had missed more days of work in the last 2 months than I had in the last 2 years. Because of my sleep problems, I was tired and irritable all the time and I felt less productive. I was running behind in my paperwork for the first time. Even when I did get work done, I felt it wasn't any good.

The physical and mental effects of depression can have a big impact on your work—both your ability to make it to work every day and to be productive. If you've spent some time away from work because of depression, returning to your workplace can be awkward. This chapter discusses how you can minimize the effects of depression on one of the important areas of your life.

LIMITING THE EFFECT OF DEPRESSION
ON THE JOB

Depressive symptoms such as sleep problems, aches and pains, fatigue, poor concentration and irritability can interfere with work functioning. You can manage most of these work problems by following some important guidelines.

It is important to try to improve organization, because concentration and memory problems are part of depression. Start each day with a list of priorities that need to be accomplished. On Sunday, or prior to the first day of your workweek, make a list of things that need to be accomplished over the week and then note things that need to be accomplished on the next day.

Pacing yourself at work is very important, because depression is associated with increased fatigue. Set reasonable deadlines, giving yourself a little longer than usual to complete projects and goals. Make sure you are taking a lunch break every day and, if you have the time at lunch, spend a half-hour in an enjoyable activity. This can include activities like taking a walk outside, talking with a trusted friend, or reading an enjoyable book. Try to limit overtime work, and make sure you are scheduling enjoyable activities on your weekends. Exercise is often helpful to clear your mind of worries, and it can improve your mood and self-esteem.

Find ways to control your anxiety and irritability in the workplace. Depression can amplify both of these emotions. If you are feeling irritable or angry with a coworker or boss, try to take a break and cool down before reapproaching the situation. If you are more anxious about a project or presentation you have to do, practice with a friend or coworker. Outline small steps to complete in order to finish the project and the time you will leave yourself for each.

WHEN DEPRESSION KEEPS YOU FROM THE JOB

If depression causes you to take time from work for more than 3 or 4 days, it is important to get help from a health professional. You may find that some professionals may be more focused than others on helping you resume your activities.

When seeking professional help, be very specific about what you want. Explain that your goal is to resume working as soon as possible; describe your work activities and explain the specific problems you are having on the job. Ask the provider if he or she can help with this problem. If your provider cannot help, ask her/him to refer you to another health professional.

There are some easy ways to judge whether the health provider is likely to help you resume activities. If you answer "yes" to the following questions then you are probably getting the assistance you need to get back to work quickly.

- Does the provider have a definite plan for my returning to work or resuming a key activity?
- Has a definite time been set for returning to work or resuming a key activity?
- Is the provider making a specific plan with either antidepressant medication or counseling to try to relieve symptoms like sleep, energy, and concentration problems?
- Is the provider willing to write a note or talk to my supervisor to speed my return to work?

If you don't feel able to return immediately to your previous level of work, you may want to offer to return part-time or start with a reduced workload. The offer will communicate to your employer that you want to work and to return as soon as possible to your prior activities. Many times, returning part-time may be better for you financially than prolonging your time off. In addition, people who return to normal activities, including work, recover faster and have fewer depression problems than those who are not working. Working regularly can take your mind off worries and help you structure your day so that the worries associated with depression will be less painful and distracting. Thus, returning to work is likely to be good for your job security, finances, self-esteem, and health.

When you return to work, the best way to protect your reputation and job security is to be conscientious about your duties and responsibilities. There may be times that you are less productive or have to miss a day, but if possible, you should make the effort to work despite your symptoms.

DEPRESSION AND THE AMERICANS WITH DISABILITIES ACT

The Americans with Disabilities Act prevents discrimination due to an illness. Therefore, employees are not allowed to discriminate against you based on your history of depression. In most cases, effective treatment will help you regain your productivity and prevent days missed from work due to depression.

Another tricky situation may arise when applying for a job. Many job applicants with a history of depression don't know whether to tell prospective employers about their condition. Experts familiar with the Americans with Disabilities Act believe that if you are physically and mentally capable of performing the job, it is best not to volunteer information about your depression. If you are positive you can handle the job, then your depression history is not relevant, and employers are not allowed to ask you about it. It is fair for employers to ask if you have any current health problems that would prevent you from undertaking the responsibilities of the job. You should answer honestly, emphasizing your ability to perform the job reliably and without risk.

If you get a job without informing your employer about your history of depression, there might well be a time when it is important to raise this issue. For instance, if a relapse occurs, you may need time to seek medical help. Depression is a medical disorder; therefore, you can state more generally that you are seeking help for a medical problem. If your work situation is supportive and under-standing, you may choose to be more specific about the problem.

Part III

TAKING CHARGE

What to Expect in This Section

Take charge by planning for

- Problems and problem solving

- Coping with or preventing relapse

- What to do if a crisis occurs

- Active participation in your daily care

FACT

People with depression experience more physical pain than those with diabetes, arthritis, or heart disease.

—*Journal of the American Medical Association*

SYMPTOMS OF DEPRESSION

Feeling irritable / Sleeping too little or too much / Loss of energy / Feeling restless / Changes in appetite / Feeling worthless / Difficulty concentrating / Thoughts of suicide / Increased anxiety / Loss of interest in enjoyable activities

CHAPTER 22

Managing Depression Day by Day

I look for signs, but depression is insidious and sneaks up
on me and snowballs. I monitor my contact with certain
people who are not supportive or positive in their own lives.
My warning signs are anxiety and not being able to sleep.

SELF-CARE ESSENTAILS

Learning to manage your depression is much like managing other things in life. You need to be able to

- Stand back and look at your problems objectively
- Set realistic goals and keep them in sight
- Look at all the possible ways of solving a problem
- Decide which solutions to try

- Evaluate which solutions are most effective and, if necessary, adjust them or try other solutions
- Reward yourself for the progress you make

Self care for depression does not mean do-it-yourself treatment. But it does mean taking personal responsibility by trying out new solutions to your problems, learning what works for you, and sticking with a plan to control depression and prevent relapse. Your first attempt to solve a problem may not work, and you may need to try something different. Developing self-care skills usually helps people with depression achieve a better quality of life.

MONITORING YOUR SYMPTOMS

How can you find out what works for you? One way is to keep track of your depressive symptoms. Monitoring your symptoms helps you learn what works for you and what doesn't. Monitoring can also be an early-warning system that will alert you quickly if you are starting to get worse.

Using the list on the opposite page, make a check mark next to the symptoms that have bothered you more often than not in the past week. This is your baseline or starting point. You will be able to assess your status by comparing this baseline number with the number of symptoms you check at any other time. There are additional copies of the symptom checklist at the back of the book.

SYMPTOM CHECKLIST FOR RECOGNIZING DEPRESSION

_____ Feeling sad, blue, irritable, or tearful

_____ Trouble sleeping or sleeping too much

_____ Fatigue or loss of energy

_____ Feeling slowed down or restless and unable to sit still

_____ Changes in appetite or weight loss or gain

_____ Loss of interest in activities you normally enjoy, such as sex

_____ Feeling worthless or guilty

_____ Feeling pessimistic or hopeless

_____ Problems concentrating or thinking

_____ Thoughts of death or suicide

_____ Aches and pains such as headache, stomachache, back pain

_____ Increased anxiety and tension or anxiety attacks

Additional copies of this checklist are located at the back of the book.

This technique of observing and writing down how you feel is called **self-monitoring.** With regular self-monitoring, you can watch your own progress in overcoming depression. Self-monitoring will also teach you to recognize the early warning signs of a depressive episode so that you can get help early and prevent your depression from coming back.

Every week, go through this list and take inventory of your symptoms. It may be easier for you to remember if you set aside a regular time to do it each week—for example, Sunday night before bed or Monday morning before work.

Alex's story:
Monitoring my symptoms has taught me about what helps me feel better. It also warns me when I'm starting to feel worse. I really believe that paying attention to how I feel and writing down what I notice can keep my depression from coming back.

DAILY MOOD RATING

Another way to check your status is to keep a log of your mood at the same time each day. Think about how you feel and assign that feeling a number from 1 (awful!) to 10 (great!).

This 1-to-10 scale may mean more to you if you think of particularly good and bad times in your life as examples at the ends of the scale. Remember the best you've ever felt in your life? That would be close to what a "10" mood feels like. Now think of the worst you've ever felt. If you believe it would be impossible to feel any worse than you did at this time of your life, give this mood a rating of "1." Now compare how you feel today with these "best" and "worst" feelings. On a scale from 1 to 10, what number describes how you feel today?

Today my mood is _____

Tomorrow and every day at about the same time, compare how you feel with how you felt the day before, and with how you felt at the best and worst times of your life. Write this number down in a small notepad or on your calendar. No one has to know what it means except you. You can use this information to determine what helps you feel better and to recognize as soon as possible when you are starting to feel worse.

CHAPTER 23

Planning for Better Living

Now that I'm starting to feel better I can see how sticking to my schedule of daily positive activities has helped me. At first I had no desire or energy to do the things my therapist suggested would help get me out of feeling so bad. I thought, "This is psychotherapy? Suggesting that I take a walk on the beach, read a magazine, spend time with friends?"

But as I have continued to take and make time for myself for enjoyable activities, I've realized how much more energy I now have to face those everyday tasks that aren't very much fun, like laundry and cleaning, and paying bills that used to really pile up. I really look forward to "my time" when I take long walks and putter in the garden.

Most important of all, I've made a habit of daily "check-ins" when I consciously go one by one through a list of depression symptoms and honestly write down which ones have been bothering me. I keep a little notebook by my bed and I've been able to see objectively the progress I've made.

I'm really committed to keeping this up long term. I never want to be taken by surprise again. I won't let this depression thing sneak up on me another time.

DEVELOPING AN ACTION PLAN

Life is full of problems. But the inevitable crises and disappointments of living can overwhelm people who are prone to depression. You may be able to use the action plan described here to keep that from happening, and to help you manage and prevent depression.

With this method, there are seven steps to solving problems:

1. Identifying the source of the difficulty
2. Pinpointing the problem
3. Listing ideas that might help solve the problem
4. Selecting one idea and trying it out
5. Assessing the results
6. Making a midcourse correction, if necessary
7. Rewarding yourself for progress

AN ACTION PLAN TO OVERCOME DEPRESSION

Denise had been recovering well from an episode of depression but began to feel that her progress had stalled. She was eager to prevent a relapse, so here's how she used an action plan in managing her depression.

Step 1: Denise identified the source of her difficulty by recognizing that she felt lonely and couldn't remember the last time she had had any fun.

Step 2: She determined that she was missing the pleasant and relaxing activities that she used to schedule all the time.

Step 3: With a friend's help, Denise made a list of all the ideas she could think of for increasing the number of pleasurable events in her life. This is her list:

- Read a juicy novel.
- Take a tap dance class.
- Join a book club.
- Rent a weekly movie and invite friends over to watch.
- Bake brownies.
- Bicycle to a park.
- Invite a friend to lunch.
- Learn Spanish.

Step 4: After looking over the list, Denise decided she would like to try biking to a park every day after work. At the park, she would sit under a tree and read a novel for half an hour.

Step 5: After 1 week, Denise assessed the results of her plan. She had gone for a bike ride only on Tuesday and Wednesday because it had rained on the other three workdays. She had enjoyed the outings, but she knew she had no desire to ride in the rain, and she was still feeling lonely.

Step 6: So Denise decided to join a cycling club where she could meet other people. At her first meeting she arranged to go for a long Saturday ride with a small group of members.

Step 7: She rewarded herself for making progress by treating herself to a massage at the end of the week.

Here's another example. Jack had started taking an antidepressant, increasing the dosage gradually as his doctor had prescribed. After a week he found himself dozing off at work and his mouth was dry for much of the time.

Step 1: Jack suspected that the medication was causing these effects, but he wasn't sure.

Step 2: He called his doctor, who confirmed that sleepiness and dry mouth were common but harmless side effects of the medicine Jack was taking.

Step 3: The doctor suggested that Jack take his antidepressant 2 or 3 hours before bedtime so that the sleepiness would wear off earlier in the morning.

Step 4: Jack also tried taking frequent short breaks at work to combat his sleepiness, and he chewed gum to relieve his dry mouth.

Step 5: Almost immediately, Jack felt more alert at work, but he still had difficulty with dry mouth.

Step 6: So he began taking a water bottle to work and found that this was more helpful than chewing gum.

Step 7: He rewarded himself for making progress by going out to a movie.

WILL AN ACTION PLAN WORK FOR YOU?

You might try out our technique on a small problem before tackling something really difficult. Don't forget Step 5, assessing the results of anything you try. You can use the worksheet on the following page to guide you through the seven steps of the action plan. Extra copies of this worksheet can be found in the back of the book.

PLANNING FOR BETTER LIVING

1. Identify the source of the difficulty.

_____

_____

2. Pinpoint the problem.

_____

_____

3. List ideas that might help solve the problem.

_____

_____

4. Select one idea and try it out.

_____

_____

5. Assess the results.

_____

_____

6. Make a midcourse correction, if necessary.

_____

_____

7. Reward yourself for progress.

_____

_____

Additional copies of this worksheet are located at the back of the book.

CHAPTER 24

Maintaining Gains and Preventing Relapse

The first time I got really depressed was just after my wife and I separated. It seemed like a natural reaction, but I was really low for months. This last time was after the end of another relationship. I thought I could handle it, but I sank even lower than the first time. I hate to say so, but I can also see a pattern of other symptoms here: getting irritable, spending more time alone, waking up in the night, missing work. Now that I'm feeling better, I want to just put it all behind me. I know, though, that I'll face other stressful times. How can I make sure I don't get into that pattern again?

CAN DEPRESSION RETURN?

Most people with depression do get better after several months, or even sooner with effective treatment. Unfortunately, your depression may return months or years later.

More than half the people who recover from an episode of major depression will have another episode someday. Three out of four people who have suffered from two or more episodes will experience another one eventually.

Reducing the Risk of Relapse

Experiencing several episodes of depression in the past does not mean you are doomed to feel depressed again. But it does mean that you need to pay attention to your moods. We have described many tools and techniques that can help you feel more in charge of depression. Maintaining your gains and preventing a recurrence will require that you use these to hone your self-care skills.

A RELAPSE PREVENTION PLAN: STRESS REDUCTION AND SELF-MONITORING

A Relapse Prevention Plan that focuses on stress reduction and self-monitoring can reduce the chance of recurrence. Your plan will permit you to intervene early, when you first begin to feel depressed and before your depression becomes severe.

KEEP DOING WHAT WORKS

Keep up successful depression-fighting strategies such as increasing your pleasurable activities and maintaining a healthy lifestyle. These strategies will help protect you against being overwhelmed by the problems we all experience.

To take inventory of the problems that can trigger your depression, and the strategies that have helped you deal with them, ask yourself:

- What are some of my everyday stress builders (for example, doing the kids' laundry, paying bills, and fighting traffic on the way to work)?
- What coping strategies have worked for me in the past (for example, taking warm baths, going for long walks with the dog, listening to music)?
- Which strategies do I think will be most useful for combating my everyday problems?
- Are these skills that I can use every day or every week?
- How can I remind myself to use these skills daily or weekly (for example, by taking deep breaths at every red light, taping a note on the bathroom door, scheduling pleasant activities on your calendar)?

The goal is to build these strategies into your day so that you can minimize the effect of life's annoyances. Try to identify three or four specific acts that help you. Be realistic about what you *can* and *will* follow up on. The more specific you can be, the more likely you are to follow through.

Sample Stress Reduction Plan

In order to prevent daily stresses from adding up, I will

1. Schedule 30 minutes for some pleasant activity every day
2. Go to the gym three times a week and sit in the gym spa after every workout
3. Go out with my buddies every Wednesday after work

Now it's your turn. List three or four things that can get you moving or lift your mood. Be specific. (What will you do? When will you do it?) Identify friends and family members who will help.

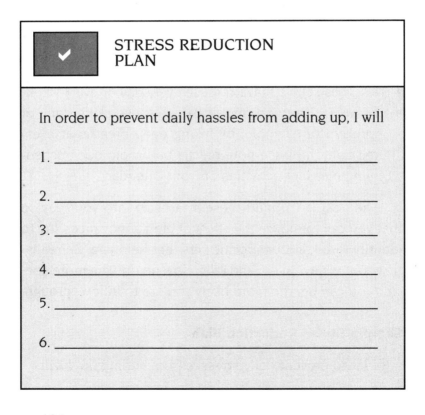

STRESS REDUCTION PLAN

In order to prevent daily hassles from adding up, I will

1. _____

2. _____

3. _____

4. _____

5. _____

6. _____

PREPARE YOURSELF FOR HIGH-RISK SITUATIONS

Major stresses are more likely than everyday annoyances to threaten your newfound stability and lead to a recurrence of depression. These might include

- Getting behind on bills or work deadlines
- Marital problems
- Separation or divorce
- Health problems
- Starting school or a new job
- Moving
- Death of a friend or family member
- Major stresses in the life of someone close to you

Prepare yourself for high-risk situations in the future by answering the following questions:

1. What are some problems and predictable stressful situations that might affect you in the future?
2. Can you do anything to make a particular stressful event less likely?
3. For those stressful situations you can't avoid, ask yourself:
   - What negative reactions (criticizing yourself, withdrawing from people) might you have in this situation?
   - How can you plan to react in a more positive way?

Think about events that have led to your depression in the past. Ask yourself, how would I react differently, knowing what I know now? The more specific you are, the better. It can be very helpful to try this approach with stressful events you know are going to happen soon, like an upcoming performance review at work.

Difficulties in your important close relationships (for example, with your spouse, partner, or children) are often the most upsetting. Significant marital or relationship troubles contribute to depression. Sometimes these issues are very painful to confront alone. One approach is to get advice and help from others, especially people who are trained to provide such help. Marital or family therapy can be the source of new perspectives and concrete solutions to your relationship problems.

Sample High-Risk Situations

1. Working too many hours of overtime

   Can you do anything to prevent it from happening?

   Yes—discuss with the boss.

   What negative reactions might you have?

   Feeling guilty for not "going the extra mile" on the job.

   Worrying that the boss or coworkers will think I'm not doing my best.

   How can you plan to react in some other way?

Remind myself that the extra money isn't worth the extra stress

Make a list of the contributions I have made to the company.

2. My ex-wife's remarriage

Can you do anything to prevent it from happening?

I wish—but not really.

What negative reactions might you have?

Comparing myself to her fiancé.

Being irritable with the kids.

How can you plan to react in some other way?

Cut myself off when I start thinking about her fiancé.

Plan a fishing trip with friends the weekend of the wedding.

My High-Risk Situations

1._____

Can you do anything to prevent it from happening?

_____

What negative reactions might you have?

_____

How can you plan to react in some other way?

_____

2._____

Can you do anything to prevent it from happening?

_____

What negative reactions might you have?

_____

How can you plan to react in some other way?

_____

WATCH FOR EARLY WARNING SIGNS

To keep future episodes of depression at bay, keep track of signals that you may be heading into depression. Paying more attention to how you're doing will mean you're less likely to be taken by surprise.

Self-Monitoring

One technique for catching depression early is regular self-monitoring. Choose a specific method for monitoring your depression level (*see the Symptom Checklist or the Daily Mood Rating, Chapter* 22) and do it regularly.

Set a specific time and place to do self-monitoring. Answering the following questions can help you decide on a regular plan for self-monitoring.

- Which method of self-monitoring (Symptom Checklist or Daily Mood Rating) is most useful for me now?
- Which method am I likely to continue doing?
- How will I remember to check up on myself daily or weekly (for example, every morning at breakfast, Sunday evening after a favorite television show)?

Personal Warning Signs

The other essential part of self-monitoring is identifying your own personal warning signs. You may have a characteristic early symptom, such as exceptionally low energy or waking up early in the morning, which tells you your depression is returning. Or you may notice some telltale pattern of thought or behavior, such as ruminating over minor mistakes, yelling when you're cut off in traffic, declining social invitations. Think about what signs will let you know you're slipping. Be specific.

You may want to ask your spouse or partner or a couple of close friends to let you know if they notice any warning signs. Sometimes other people are aware of such changes before you are.

Sandra's story:

When I thought about it, I realized that I tend to listen to certain kinds of music when I'm feeling down. I mentioned this to my boyfriend, and he jumped right on it. He said there's one CD that's a "dead give-away." If he hears it through the apartment door, he knows it will be a rough evening. Now that I am feeling better, I can even laugh about it. I got out the CD and wrote myself a note inside the cover: "Before listening, find and read your Relapse Prevention Plan." Actually, I doubt I'll get as far as opening it. Just thinking about it will be enough to get me to check up on my mood.

Sample Self-Monitoring Plan

I will monitor my symptoms using (Symptom Checklist, Daily Mood Rating)

<u>Symptom Checklist</u>

When: <u>On Fridays after work</u>

Where: <u>At my desk</u>

Personal Warning Signs—I'll look for other signs of depression if I find myself

1. <u>Making up excuses for missing a softball game</u>
2. <u>Not getting dressed before noon on weekend</u>
3. _____

Now it's your turn.

✔	**SELF-MONITORING PLAN**

I will monitor my symptoms using (Symptom Check-list, Daily Mood Rating)

_____

When: _____

Where: _____

Personal Warning Signs—I'll look for other signs of depression if I find myself

1. _____

2. _____

3. _____

4. _____

HAVE A "BOOSTER PLAN" IN CASE
YOU START TO SLIP

Your self-monitoring plan will alert you early if your depression is starting to return. If you do notice your mood start to drop or see other warning signs of depression, you'll be prepared to take action.

The first step is to return to your Stress Reduction Plan. Have you been taking care of yourself as well as you had planned? If not, what steps should you take during the next week to get back on track? The next step is to turn to a Booster Plan of extra things you need to do if you start slipping. An effective booster plan should be flexible. You're more likely to be successful if you can call on reinforcements from a number of directions.

Possible components of a Booster Plan include

- **Activation.** When you feel like doing nothing, do something—something rewarding. Plan an activity for each day, and be specific. Include others in your plans; it's harder to back out of a commitment you've made to someone else.
- **Support.** Identify friends or family members you can call on for some extra support. It may feel awkward to ask, but the best approach is a direct one: "I've really been feeling down for the last few weeks, and I need some help getting going. Can we schedule times to get together over the next few weeks? I need to do this, so don't let me make excuses and back out later."

- **Antidepressants or Psychotherapy.** If treatment for depression (either medications or psychotherapy) has been helpful for you in the past, your booster plan should probably include a suggestion that you consider re-contacting your doctor or therapist. If you started to notice a return of depression soon after stopping treatment, this may be an indication that re-starting treatment would be a good idea. If you've noticed signs of depression returning while you're still receiving treatment (either medications or psychotherapy), be sure to discuss this with your doctor or therapist. *Chapter 7 of this book, "When Is Treatment Finished," includes more specific information about how long you should continue treatment for depression.*

Sample Booster Plan

If I notice depression returning, I will

1. <u>Do something outdoors on my way home from work every day</u>

2. <u>Call Jessie, Pat, and Reggie to set up some time together over the weekend</u>

3. <u>Call my brother and my sister at least twice a week until things get better</u>

4. <u>Call Dr. Reynolds about adjusting the medication (phone: 555-5555)</u>

Now it's your turn.

My Booster Plan

If I notice depression returning, I will

1. _____

2. _____

3. _____

4. _____

PULLING IT ALL TOGETHER

Now you have filled in a rough draft of your Relapse Prevention Plan. Keep a copy of your plan in a place where you can refer to it each time you do your self-monitoring.

You may also want to give blank copies (located in the back of this book) to a couple of close friends or family members. You may be surprised at how helpful they can be at identifying personal warning signs that you didn't think of. They may also be willing to help you stick with your Stress Reduction Plan.

STRESS REDUCTION PLAN

In order to prevent daily hassles from adding up, I will

1. _____

2. _____

3. _____

4. _____

High-Risk Situations

#1 _____

Can you do anything to prevent it from happening?

_____

What negative reactions might you have?

_____

How can you plan to react in some other way?

_____

#2 _____

Can you do anything to prevent it from happening?

_____

What negative reactions might you have?

_____

How can you plan to react in some other way?

_____

SELF-MONITORING PLAN

I will monitor my symptoms using (Symptom Checklist, Daily Mood Rating)

_____

When: _____

Where: _____

Personal Warning Signs—I'll look for other signs of depression if I find myself

1. _____

2. _____

3. _____

4. _____

Booster Plan
If I notice depression returning, I will

1. _____

2. _____

3. _____

4. _____

Additional copies of both worksheets can be found in the back of the book.

CHAPTER 25

Living Your Plan

It helps that I know more now about my own normal behavior and about the signs of depression. I have a better sense of what I can expect, and I'm better at monitoring myself. I also have less contact with morose people, I'm willing to go to counseling if that seems necessary, and I trust family and friends and coworkers to comment if they see signs that I'm getting depressed again.

SOME CHANGES MAY BE NECESSARY

Managing and preventing depression can mean some major changes in your life. You may have already made significant adjustments in your usual ways of thinking and behaving. For example, you may be taking an antidepressant every day, a big step for many people. And preventing relapse may involve scheduling time at least once a week for self-monitoring and review.

If you're like most people, you'll slip up at times. You'll drift back toward old patterns, miss a self-monitoring appointment here and there, and sometimes even forget your medication.

Fortunately, your long-term success at beating depression doesn't depend on keeping to your plan perfectly. It does depend on paying attention when you stray from it. But don't condemn yourself. Punishing yourself every time you slip up will not prevent lapses. It just makes you less likely to admit them to yourself. Try a different approach. Ask yourself, "How can I prevent this or catch it sooner next time?" You have lots of time to practice.

Your family and friends may need a period of adjustment, too. You feel different, and you're likely to act different. You may be more assertive about what you want or need to do. Planning your time and looking out for yourself will sometimes affect other people's plans as well.

Most of the changes will be good for everyone, but friends or family members may sometimes misinterpret what you do or take it personally. If you stand up for yourself, they may think you're angry with them. If you aren't as willing to let them set the agenda, they may wonder what they've done to provoke this new reaction from you.

If you notice this sort of reaction from people close to you, honesty is the best policy. Let them know that you've been working hard at taking better care of yourself, spending more time having fun, avoiding self-criticism, increasing your self-confidence. Explain that you'll need to experiment with different ways of doing things. Most important, ask for their help in sticking to the worthwhile changes you've made in your life.

SOMETIMES IT'S WISE TO BLOW YOUR COVER

In preparing your Relapse Prevention Plan, you probably noticed several characteristic patterns that are part of your depression. For example, you may typically cut down on enjoyable activities and withdraw from friends, family, and coworkers.

You may also have noticed how you cover your tracks, slipping into a depressed pattern without letting anyone know. For example, you might tell people that you have the flu or that you're too busy to see them. Or you might just stop returning phone calls.

Perhaps it's time to blow your cover. Choose a few friends or family members you can depend on. Talk with them about the ways you withdraw when you're feeling depressed. You might be surprised: they may know your excuses as well as you do.

Explain how you'd like them to respond next time they notice you slipping, and give them permission to call you on it. You might even tell them exactly what kind of response would be most helpful to you.

Jane's story:

When depression is coming on, I put off tasks at work and around the house. If this goes on for a few weeks, I get behind and start to feel like I'm never going to catch up. I talked to my husband and my closest friend at work about this. Now they keep an eye out for this pattern. Once a month or so, one of them will ask me how it's going. When I start to get in a rut, I know it's time to get help before the depression is severe.

UPDATE YOUR RELAPSE PREVENTION PLAN

You will probably revise your relapse prevention strategies over time. You may change your plans about medication, for example. Or you may find new activities to reduce your tension level. You'll undoubtedly be faced with new problems and stresses, just like everybody else.

Review and update your Relapse Prevention Plan regularly. Follow-up visits to your doctor or counselor can be an ideal time for review. Bring your plan to the visit. After you and your doctor have discussed how you're doing, write a new plan for the next few months. If you're not visiting a doctor regularly, update your plan at least every 6 months.

STAY CONFIDENT, BUT BE PREPARED

When you're feeling better, it's easy to forget about the things you did to get there. You may feel so good that you're tempted to stop taking your antidepressant without discussing it with your doctor. Or you may feel you can stop scheduling regular pleasant and relaxing activities because your energy level has improved so much.

You don't want to ignore the possibility of slipping back into depression, but going to the other extreme can also be a bad idea. The key is to concentrate on what you can do to stay healthy. Having a specific plan of action is a way to avoid getting mired in fruitless worry about your future.

We hope this book has helped you learn more about depression and ways in which you can participate fully in your own health care. You may want to refer back to certain sections periodically. As you recover, information that seems confusing or unimportant now may become more useful.

We wish you well.

A Primer on Antidepressants

There are several different kinds of antidepressants. All of them are effective in relieving the symptoms of depression, but none works for everybody who is depressed. Different types of antidepressants also tend to have different kinds of side effects. In the lists below, the first name is the antidepressant's scientific or generic name, followed in parentheses by its brand, or proprietary, name. We list typical doses for each medication, but doses vary widely from person to person. Doses are typically lower for people over age 60 or those with a chronic medical illness. All of the drugs in this section should be taken according to the dose and manner prescribed by your doctor.

SEROTONIN REUPTAKE INHIBITORS (SRIs)

The newest antidepressants have quickly become quite popular. Known as selective serotonin reuptake inhibitors

(SRIs), they work by increasing the amount of the neuro-transmitter serotonin available in the brain. SRIs are chemically unrelated to the tricyclics and are considered to have fewer and more tolerable side effects than many of the older antidepressants.

Common SRIs

Citalopram (Celexa): Common side effects include nausea, gastrointestinal irritability, headaches, jitteriness, decreased ability to achieve orgasm, and insomnia. Switching to a different antidepressant is required in 5%–15% of patients.

Fluoxetine (Prozac): Fluoxetine was the first, and is still the best known, of the SRIs. Common side effects include nausea, gastrointestinal irritability, headaches, jitteriness, decreased ability to achieve orgasm, and insomnia. Switching to a different antidepressant is required in 5%–15% of patients.

Fluvoxamine (Luvox): Common side effects include nausea, gastrointestinal irritability, headaches, jitteriness, decreased ability to achieve orgasm, and insomnia. Switching to a different antidepressant is required in 5%–15% of patients.

Paroxetine (Paxil): Common side effects include nausea, gastrointestinal irritability, headaches, jitteriness, decreased ability to achieve orgasm, and insomnia. Switching to a different antidepressant is required in 5%–15% of patients.

Sertraline (Zoloft): Common side effects include nausea, gastrointestinal irritability, headaches, jitteriness, decreased ability to achieve orgasm, and insomnia. Switching to a different antidepressant is required in 5%–15% of patients.

OTHER NEWER ANTIDEPRESSANTS

Bupropion (Wellbutrin): This medication is different from most other antidepressants; it may work by increasing the action of dopamine, another neurotransmitter. Common side effects include jitteriness, nausea, and sleep disturbance. Because large doses at a single time can slightly increase the risk of seizures or convulsions, it is usually taken two or three times per day.

Mirtazapine (Remeron): This antidepressant also increases the action of serotonin and norepinephrine, but it does not have as frequent sexual side effects as the SRI medications described above. Common side effects include sedation, dizziness, weight gain, and dry mouth.

Nefazadone (Serzone): Another new antidepressant, nefazodone also acts by increasing the action of serotonin. Nefazodone appears to have fewer sexual side effects than the SRI medications described above and is less likely to cause jitteriness. Common side effects include nausea, gastrointestinal irritability, headache, jitteriness, and sedation. Switching to a different antidepressant is required in 5%–15% of patients.

Venlafaxine (Effexor): This is one of the newest antidepressants. It increases the amount of both serotonin and norepinephrine available at nerve synapses in the brain. Venlafaxine sometimes causes dry mouth, dizziness, constipation, urinary hesitancy, and blurred vision. It can also cause sexual side effects, but probably does so less often than most of the other SRI medications. In about 5% of patients, venlafaxine can raise blood pressure.

TRICYCLIC (OR HETEROCYCLIC) ANTIDEPRESSANTS

Tricyclics, developed in the late 1950s and early 1960s, were the first antidepressants. Most of them work by increasing the amount of the neurotransmitters norepinephrine and (to a lesser extent) serotonin available at *synapses*, the tiny spaces between nerve cells, in the brain. As a group, the tricyclics tend to produce the following side effects: dry mouth, constipation, hesitancy in urinating, blurred vision, sleepiness, weight gain, dizziness when changing quickly from a lying or sitting position to standing up (postural hypotension), and increased heart rate or pulse rate. For most people these side effects are tolerable, but in about 10%–20% of cases a switch to a different antidepressant is required.

Commonly Prescribed Tricyclics

Amitriptyline (Elavil): One of the earliest antidepressants. Common side effects include dry mouth, constipation, urinary hesitancy, blurred vision, sedation, weight gain, postural hypotension, and increased heart or pulse rate.

Desipramine (Norpramin): This drug's side effects tend to be less troublesome than those of the older tricyclics such as imipramine or sinequan, but they are similar in kind: dry mouth, constipation, urinary hesitancy, blurred vision, sedation, weight gain, postural hypotension, increased heart rate and rash. For most patients these side effects are tolerable, but in 5%–15% of cases a switch to a different medication is required.

Imipramine (Tofranil): One of the first tricyclics. Common side effects include dry mouth, constipation, urinary hesitancy, blurred vision, sedation, weight gain, postural hypotension, and increased heart or pulse rate.

Nortriptyline (Pamelor): Nortriptyline's side effects are less severe than those of most other tricyclic antidepressants. Side effects include sleepiness, dry mouth, constipation, urinary hesitancy, blurred vision, weight gain, postural hypotension, and increased heart or pulse rate. In 5%-15% of patients, side effects require switching medication.

Protriptyline (Vivactil): Protriptyline causes increased energy and, as a result, is usually taken in the morning. In addition to the usual side effects associated with tricyclics, protriptyline can cause jitteriness.

(Doxepin) Sinequan: Doxepin is one of the antidepressants most likely to cause sedation. Other common side effects

include dry mouth, constipation, urinary hesitancy, blurred vision, weight gain, postural hypotension, and increased heart or pulse rate.

Newer Tricyclics

Amoxapine (Asendin): Amoxapine is not usually recommended except for depressed patients with psychotic symptoms, such as hallucinations or delusions. It increases the amount of norepinephrine and (to a lesser extent) serotonin available at nerve synapses in the brain. Possible side effects include those common to the tricyclics. In rare cases, it can cause long-term problems with muscle twitching or spasms.

Maprotiline (Ludiomil): This medication increases the amount of the neurotransmitter norepinephrine available at nerve synapses in the brain. Its side effects are the usual ones seen with tricyclic antidepressants. For most patients its side effects are mild to moderate, but in 5% to 15% of cases they require changing medication. Ludiomil does slightly increase the risk of seizures or convulsions.

Trazodone (Desyrel): Trazodone has been available for about 15 years. It increases the amount of serotonin available at synapses in the brain. Side effects include sedation, postural hypotension, and weight gain. A more severe (but rare) side effect is priapism, a prolonged erection. Because of its sedating properties, trazodone is sometimes used in low doses for the treatment of insomnia. Most patients can tolerate its side effects, but about 5%–15% switch to another antidepressant.

MAO INHIBITORS

Monoamine oxidase (MAO) inhibitors affect mood by increasing the amount of the neurotransmitters norepinephrine, epinephrine, and serotonin available at synapses in the brain. MAO inhibitors are often prescribed when other antidepressants have not been successful. Patients taking MAO inhibitors must avoid certain foods, especially those containing tyramine, a chemical that helps regulate blood pressure. Tyramine is found in foods such as bananas, herring, chicken livers, avocados, and eggplant, as well as in beer and wine and in aged foods like dried sausage and cheese. Over-the-counter diet, cold, and asthma medications, among others, are also off limits when taking most MAO inhibitors. Check with your doctor or pharmacist for a complete list of things to avoid if you are taking one of the drugs in this class.

Common MAO Inhibitors

Phenelzine (Nardil): Common side effects include fatigue, weakness, postural hypotension, restlessness, tremors, dry mouth, constipation, urination difficulties, blurred vision, and "sweet tooth."

Tranylcypromine (*Parnate*): Common side effects include fatigue, weakness, postural hypotension, restlessness, tremors, dry mouth, constipation, urination difficulties, blurred vision and "sweet tooth."

RESOURCE GUIDE

ORGANIZATIONS

Call, write, or check the internet for information and referrals, and to learn about local chapters and support groups.

American Psychiatric Association
Division of Public Affairs
Suite 500
1400 K St., NW
Washington, DC 20005
Free pamphlets are available
1-888-357-7924 or 202-682-6119
Fax: 202-682-6850
www.psych.org

Depression After Delivery, Inc.
91 E. Somerset St.
Raritan, NJ 018869
1-800-944-4773
www.depressionafterdelivery.com

Depression Awareness, Recognition and Treatment Program (D/ART)
National Institute of Mental Health
5600 Fishers Lane, Room 10-85
Rockville, MD 20857
1-800-421-4211 or 301-443-4140
Fax: 301-443-4045
www.nimh.nih.gov/dart/

National Alliance for the Mentally Ill

Colonial Place Three,
2107 Wilson Blvd., Suite 300
Arlington, VA 22201-3042
1-800-950-6264 (Help Line)
703-524-7600 (Business Line)
Fax: 703-524-9094
www.nami.org

National Depressive and Manic-Depressive Association

730 N. Franklin St., Suite 501
Chicago, IL 60610-7204
1-800-826-3632 or 312-642-0049
Fax: 312-642-7243
www.ndmda.org

National Foundation for Depressive Illness

PO Box 2257
New York, NY 10116-2257
1-800-239-1265
www.depression.org

National Mental Health Association

1021 Prince St.
Alexandria, VA 22314-2971
1-800-969-6642 or 703-684-7722
Fax: 703-684-5968
www.nmha.org

BOOKS

Control Your Depression by Peter M. Lewinsohn, PhD, Ricardo Munoz, PhD, Mary Ann Youngren, PhD, and Antonette M. Zeiss, PhD; Simon and Trade paperbacks, NY, 1992. To order, call: 1-888-866-6631.

The Depression Workbook: A Guide for Living with Depression and Manic Depression by Mary Ellen Copeland, Matthew Mckay, Ph.D., and Mary Liz Riddle, New Harbinger Publications, Oakland, CA, 2001. To order, call 1-800-748-6273.

Feeling Good: The New Mood Therapy by David D. Burns and Aaron T. Beck, Morrow, William & Company, NY, 1999. To obtain a list of distributors, check the publisher's website, www.harpercollins.com.

The Feeling Good Handbook by David D. Burns, M.D.; Penguin USA, NY, 1999. To order, call 1-800-526-0275.

The Noonday Demon: An Atlas of Depression by Andrew Solomon, Simon and Schuster Trade, NY, 2001. To order, call 1-888-866-6631.

On the Edge of Darkness: Conversations about Conquering Depression by Kathy Cronkite; Bantam Dell Publishing Group, NY, 1995. To order, call 1-800-733-3000 or 1-800-726-0600.

Silencing the Self: Women and Depression by Dana Crowley Jack; HarperTrade, NY, 1993. To obtain a list of distributors, check the publisher's website, www.harpercollins.com.

Winter Blues: Seasonal Affective Disorder—What It Is and How to Overcome It by Norman Rosenthal, M.D.; Guilford Publications, Inc., NY, 1998. To order, call 1-800-365-7006.

To Be or Not to Be—On Hormone Replacement Therapy: A Workbook to Help You Explore Your Options, originally developed by the Group Health Cooperative Center for Health Studies and the Centers for Disease Control and Prevention. Currently available through the Federal Consumer Information Center (FCIC), 1-888-8PUEBLO.

The Coping with Depression Course: A Psychoeducational Invention for Unipolar Depression* by P.M. Lewinsohn, D. O Antoniuccio, J.L. Steinmetz-Breckenridge, and L. Teri; Castalia Publishing Company, Eugene, OR, 1984.

Leader's Manual for Parent Groups: Adolescent Coping with Depression Course* by P.M. Lewinsohn, P. Rhode, H. Hops, and G. Clarke; Castalia Publishing Company, Eugene, OR, 1990.

Leader's Manual for Adolescent Groups: Adolescent Coping with Depression Course* by P.M. Lewinsohn and H. Hops; Castalia Publishing Company, Eugene, OR, 1990.

The Prevention of Depression: Research and Practice* by R.F. Munoz, Y. Ying, E.J. Perez-Stable, and J. Miranda; Johns Hopkins University Press, Baltimore, MD, 1993.

I Can If I Want To* by Arnold Lazarus, Ph.D., and Allen Fay, M.D.; William, Morrow and Company, NY, 1992.

---

* These books were out of print as of February 2002. You may be able to find them in your local library or at a used bookstore.

SYMPTOM CHECKLIST FOR RECOGNIZING DEPRESSION

_____ Feeling sad, blue, irritable, or tearful

_____ Trouble sleeping or sleeping too much

_____ Fatigue or loss of energy

_____ Feeling slowed down or restless and unable to sit still

_____ Changes in appetite or weight loss or gain

_____ Loss of interest in activities you normally enjoy, such as sex

_____ Feeling worthless or guilty

_____ Feeling pessimistic or hopeless

_____ Problems concentrating or thinking

_____ Thoughts of death or suicide

_____ Aches and pains such as headache, stomachache, back pain

_____ Increased anxiety and tension or anxiety attacks

SYMPTOM CHECKLIST FOR RECOGNIZING DEPRESSION

_____ Feeling sad, blue, irritable, or tearful

_____ Trouble sleeping or sleeping too much

_____ Fatigue or loss of energy

_____ Feeling slowed down or restless and unable to sit still

_____ Changes in appetite or weight loss or gain

_____ Loss of interest in activities you normally enjoy, such as sex

_____ Feeling worthless or guilty

_____ Feeling pessimistic or hopeless

_____ Problems concentrating or thinking

_____ Thoughts of death or suicide

_____ Aches and pains such as headache, stomachache, back pain

_____ Increased anxiety and tension or anxiety attacks

MAKING TIME FOR ENJOYMENT

1. What are some pleasurable activities you have enjoyed in the past?

_____

_____

_____

2. What would be enjoyable to do right now?

_____

_____

_____

3. What social activities could you plan to arrange this week?

_____

_____

_____

4. What small thing could you do today that would be an accomplishment for you?

_____

_____

_____

MAKING TIME FOR ENJOYMENT

1. What are some pleasurable activities you have enjoyed in the past?

_____

_____

_____

2. What would be enjoyable to do right now?

_____

_____

_____

3. What social activities could you plan to arrange this week?

_____

_____

_____

4. What small thing could you do today that would be an accomplishment for you?

_____

_____

_____

PLANNING FOR
BETTER LIVING

1. Identify the source of the difficulty.

_____

_____

2. Pinpoint the problem.

_____

_____

3. List ideas that might help solve the problem.

_____

_____

4. Select one idea and try it out.

_____

_____

5. Assess the results.

_____

_____

6. Make a midcourse correction, if necessary.

_____

_____

7. Reward yourself for progress.

_____

_____

PLANNING FOR
BETTER LIVING

1. Identify the source of the difficulty.

_____

_____

2. Pinpoint the problem.

_____

_____

3. List ideas that might help solve the problem.

_____

_____

4. Select one idea and try it out.

_____

_____

5. Assess the results.

_____

_____

6. Make a midcourse correction, if necessary.

_____

_____

7. Reward yourself for progress.

_____

_____

STRESS REDUCTION PLAN

In order to prevent daily hassles from adding up, I will

1. _____

2. _____

3. _____

4. _____

High-Risk Situations

#1 _____

Can you do anything to prevent it from happening?

_____

What negative reactions might you have?

_____

How can you plan to react in some other way?

_____

#2 _____

Can you do anything to prevent it from happening?

_____

What negative reactions might you have?

_____

How can you plan to react in some other way?

_____

STRESS REDUCTION
PLAN

In order to prevent daily hassles from adding up, I will

1. _____

2. _____

3. _____

4. _____

High-Risk Situations

#1 _____

Can you do anything to prevent it fromhappening?

_____

What negative reactions might you have?

_____

How can you plan to react in some other way?

_____

#2 _____

Can you do anything to prevent it from happening?

_____

What negative reactions might you have?

_____

How can you plan to react in some other way?

_____

SELF-MONITORING PLAN

I will monitor my symptoms using (Symptom Checklist, Daily Mood Rating)

_____

When: _____

Where: _____

Personal Warning Signs—I'll look for other signs of depression if I find myself

1. _____

2. _____

3. _____

4. _____

Booster Plan
If I notice depression returning, I will

1. _____

2. _____

3. _____

4. _____

SELF-MONITORING PLAN

I will monitor my symptoms using (Symptom Check-list, Daily Mood Rating)

_____

When: _____

Where: _____

Personal Warning Signs—I'll look for other signs of depression if I find myself

1. _____

2. _____

3. _____

4. _____

Booster Plan
If I notice depression returning, I will

1. _____

2. _____

3. _____

4. _____

INDEX